10 - 28 - 85

Genes, Blood, and Courage

And if He closes before you
The ways and passes all
He'll show you a hidden pathway
Which nobody has known

Jalal-ud-din-Rumi
Eleventh-century Persian mystic

Genes, Blood, and Courage

A Boy Called Immortal Sword

DAVID G. NATHAN

THE BELKNAP PRESS OF
HARVARD UNIVERSITY PRESS
Cambridge, Massachusetts
London, England
1995

Library of Congress Cataloging-in-Publication Data

Nathan, David G., 1929–
Genes, blood, and courage : a boy called Immortal Sword /
David G. Nathan.
p.   cm.
Includes bibliographical references and index.
ISBN 0-674-34473-1
1. Thalassemia—Research—Methodology.
2. Thalassemia—Case studies.
3. Thalassemia—Molecular aspects.
RC641.7.T5N38 1995
362.1'96152'0092—dc20
[B]
95-6080

Preface

THIS BOOK is a medical detective story that centers on one patient, Dayem Saif, who inherited a severe anemia called thalassemia. This disease is not as well known in the United States as hemophilia, sickle cell anemia, or cystic fibrosis, but it is one of the commonest inherited disorders in the world, particularly along the shores of the Mediterranean Sea, the rivers of the Middle East, the swampy areas of India, and the valleys of the Far East and Southeast Asia. I have chosen to write about a patient with this particular disease because over the past twenty-five years thalassemia has provided medical researchers with an unparalleled opportunity to plumb the depths of the structure and function of human genes.

An entirely new force in medical care called molecular medicine is about to bring tremendous advances in the rational diagnosis, prevention, and treatment of inherited diseases, and even of acquired diseases such as cancer. Patients like Dayem and their physicians have been in the vanguard of these advances in clinical and basic research. This book is a chronicle of these many successes as well as the story of a patient. Into Dayem's fascinating case history I try to weave the clinical and laboratory achievements that have led to what is now known as the genetic revolution. A worldwide scientific effort has heightened our awareness of human genes and their connection to disease. Parts of this book deal with the training and development of some of the physician-scientists who have participated in this exciting quest and with the conflicts in research policy that have arisen along the way. Although I have deliberately emphasized the accomplishments of researchers whom I have known or with whom I have worked, the reader must understand that knowledge of thalassemia and other genetic diseases is the work of many hands around the world. My story is just one aspect of a much bigger picture.

When I began my work on thalassemia, next to nothing was understood of its genetic basis. Today we know the precise molecular causes of nearly every case of the disease. By combining accurate prenatal diagnosis with selective abortion, we can prevent it. Now we are working on ways to correct this inherited defect that so damages the red cells of its victims. In the meanwhile, new approaches to treatment have sustained the life of these patients while they await a fundamental cure. Bone marrow transplantation has already cured many of them, and gene transfer therapy may eventually free many others from this terrible disease.

In Dayem Saif's case, there have been great triumphs, and there have been moments of terrible defeat. Dayem has been courageous and determined, but he is maddeningly rebellious, and I have had many periods of fear that I would lose him. Through it all, Dayem has been transformed from a tiny, misshapen victim of profound anemia, heart failure, and multiple fractures to an energetic businessman and *bon vivant*.

To protect the privacy of Dayem and his family, I have given him an Arabic pseudonym derived from the English interpretation of his actual Arabic name, which translates to "Immortal Sword." I have also altered his family history somewhat. Aside from these changes, I have tried to tell this story exactly as I have recorded it over the past twenty-five years.

I began thinking of this book in the mid-1970s, when I had an opportunity to serve on Harvard University Press's board of faculty advisers, a body quaintly known as the Board of Syndics. My job was to review books with a medical slant. Arthur Rosenthal, then the Director of the Press, often asked me to write about thalassemia. I demurred because I was too busy working on the illness in the laboratory and clinic. Before I decided to put pen to paper I wanted to be certain that Dayem would grow to independence and that the basic science that underpins his care had arrived at a point where it could be clearly explained. I write this now while awaiting the next big step, the actual molecular correction of his defect. That could happen within the next two decades. If it does, thousands of patients with inherited diseases will be the joyful beneficiaries.

Arthur, who has since moved to a senior publishing role in New York, introduced me to my splendid agent, Jill Kneerim, of The Palmer and Dodge Agency in Boston. Jill understands my commitment to my patient Dayem, to the ultimate solution to his disease, and to a life in academic medicine. Not only has she taught me about the business of writing, she has also taught me about the art as well. Jill, in turn, introduced me to Ruth Hapgood, a fine editor who guided me with firm diplomacy when the first draft was completed and a book began to take shape.

Barbara Culliton, a master science writer, has given me much of her precious time, helping me to smooth out rough scientific passages while urging me to make clear statements with few words. Richard Preston, a wonderful writer and friend, guided me in the early phase of the book. My friend and tennis partner Derek Bok devoted many hours to the task, helping me to prune away tendentious passages. Stuart H. Orkin, Sir David Weatherall, and Fred S. Rosen carefully combed the text for errors of fact as well as style. If any errors remain, they are mine. Finally, my book was turned over to Harvard University Press, where Michael Fisher and Susan Wallace Boehmer made important suggestions that have improved the text and the illustrations—the latter so well prepared by Kathy Stern (with assistance on figure 1 from Robert Rubin and Drs. James Jandl and Orah Platt). Susan is a remarkable manuscript editor; working with her during the final stages of this project has been a joy. I hope my friendly critics are finally pleased; I remain grateful to all of them.

As work on thalassemia continues and new ideas emerge that we would not have even considered a few decades ago, I understand even more firmly how fortunate I am to be a member of a small group of academic physicians privileged to explore new ways to combat old and new illnesses. Ever since I left the National

Cancer Institute three and a half decades ago, I have been supported by grants from the National Institutes of Health, the March of Dimes, the American Heart Association, the American Cancer Society, the Cooley's Anemia Foundation, the Medical Foundation, Genetics Institute, the Hellenic Women's Club, Inc., the Charles H. Hood Foundation, the Lucille P. Mackey Charitable Trust, and the Dyson Foundation to work on projects that continuously excite and challenge me. I should also like to acknowledge the contribution to Children's Hospital research provided by the Howard Hughes Medical Institute's unit and each of its investigators. All of this support has enabled me to work in a wonderful children's hospital and cancer institute embedded in a great medical school, where I am surrounded by some of the brightest clinical investigators and basic scientists in the world. I am particularly indebted to Children's Hospital, the Dana-Farber Cancer Institute, and Harvard Medical School for providing me with an environment that fosters my research and my commitment to children with inherited diseases, and to Dr. Frederick Lovejoy, the attending staff, and the house staff in pediatrics at Children's Hospital, who care so wonderfully for our patients.

I am also fortunate to remain entrusted with the training of many younger clinical investigators, some of whose contributions have already eclipsed my own. I hold a particularly warm affection for the fellows and staff of the Division of Hematology and Oncology at Children's Hospital and the Dana-Farber Cancer Institute, with whom I have worked productively for nearly thirty years. In that division, of which I was the chief for twenty years, I learned the joy and inspiration that accrues to those who are privileged to teach and train. Long after my papers and books are forgotten, their work and their students will be carrying on the search for better treatment. That is a legacy that makes me very proud.

Most important, the patients who seek my advice have presented fascinating problems. They and their families are remarkable people who understand that we must move ahead with caution. They never press me to go beyond my own borders of safety, yet they are more eager for progress than I can ever be. They want to see themselves or their children rid of the burdens they carry, and they trust me to do my best for them. By describing Dayem and some of my other patients with thalassemia, I have tried to thank them for that trust.

There comes a moment when a book must be taken out of one's mind and set on paper. The Bellagio Study Center of the Rockefeller Foundation gave me five precious weeks of tranquility and concentration during which the initial draft emerged. I am very grateful to the Bellagio staff and to Derek and Sissela Bok, who urged me to apply to become a scholar-in-residence there.

Despite computers and word-processing programs, books require technical expertise. I have had wonderful technical assistance from Janet Cameron, Amy Craig, Cathryn Lantigua, and Allison Pedroza. Cathy has provided excellent editorial assistance as well, and she and Janet, together with our Department Manager, Sally Andrews, have managed my professional life so competently that I have time to think and write.

This book required the enthusiastic support and participation of Dayem and his family. We began as doctor and patient and became very good friends. I thank them and all of my patients and their families for the honor of serving them.

Finally and most importantly I have been blessed for more than four decades by the companionship of my wife, Jean, who has read every page of this book a dozen times and has encouraged me to pursue this and every other project that I have undertaken. I thank her, my three children, and my six grandchildren for being with me and for making the insufficient time that I have with them so loving. This book is dedicated to Jean for our forty-fifth anniversary.

Contents

The First Meeting 1

Killer or Savior 18

Seduced by Thalassemia 38

Grasping Opportunities 59

Hard Choices 77

Iron Overload 98

A New Face 122

Banned in Boston 135

The Recombinant DNA Scare 155

Failing Genes 173

From Drugs to Gene Therapy 192

Closing In 211

Celebration and Reflection 228

Families, Patients, and Doctors 243

Further Reading 250

Glossary 251

Index 268

The First Meeting

I WAS STUNNED when I first saw him. Dayem Saif had been referred to me by his Portuguese pediatrician in the fall of 1968, because of my particular interest in the blood disorder he had inherited. In our pediatric hematology clinic at Children's Hospital in Boston, we specialize in caring for children with complicated blood diseases.

Dayem was then a six-year-old with the stature of an average boy of two. His belly protruded between the buttons of his finely embroidered linen shirt, yet his elegant blue woolen shorts and matching jacket with brass buttons gave him the appearance of a doll-like English Public School boy. His legs looked like twigs, and on his tiny feet he wore baby shoes. As he moved carefully down the long corridor of the clinic, hand in hand with his mother, I could hear his noisy breathing ten feet away.

Dayem's skin was dark yet pasty, a result of his Syrian and Iranian lineage and severe anemia. His massive head, with its carefully combed sun-bleached hair, seemed barely supported by his frail neck and shoulders. His face was terribly misshapen. An enormous bulging forehead, upper teeth pushed forward by a swollen upper jaw, and a receding lower jaw gave him the appearance of a highly cerebral gargoyle.

This tiny child, his breathing made even noisier and faster by the short walk from the waiting area to the examination room, calmly gazed about the hallway with a practiced look, as though he had been in similar surroundings many times, in many places, and was accustomed to doctors, nurses, and the usual paraphernalia of a hospital clinic. When his eyes turned to look at me, however, a ravishing smile lit up his face. Bowing slightly, he put out his hand to greet me, and as I bent from the waist and gently shook his hand, I felt that I had known him for years. We stood together while I introduced myself to his parents and brothers.

I was accustomed to the sight of children with thalassemia, a serious inherited anemia that is one of the commonest diseases in the world. Thalassa refers, in Greek, to the Mediterranean Sea, and the rest of the name comes from *haima,* the Greek word for blood. So the name of the disease suggests that it is a blood disease found among people who live near the Mediterranean Sea. The group of hematologists in our clinic were caring for several children with this affliction, most of whom had come to us from the Italian and Greek communities of New England. Were it not for the treatment programs available in hospitals like ours, these children would have shared Dayem's stunted growth and facial deformity.

The mothers of these children usually did not attract particular attention at our hospital. Their careworn faces and anxious eyes, surrounded by dark circles of distress and fatigue, were typical of mothers whose children suffer from chronic disease. They are usually good mothers, filled with concern for the fate of their children, but also preoccupied by the financial crisis that assails most American families when long-term illness strikes. The dual assaults of fear that a child may die and worry that medical costs may wipe out the family savings or force them from their homes leave many of them exhausted.

In contrast, Dayem's mother had attracted every eye in the clinic. She had a warm and magnificent beauty and a sense of style that left all of us feeling drab and provincial. Her tawny hair was parted in the middle and fell just to the side of her large hazel eyes. She wore gold earrings that matched her necklace and bracelet. Her tailored tan linen suit—carefully chosen to set off her light complexion and slender figure—was accented by a silk scarf casually knotted around her neck.

Part of the aura of calm beauty that surrounded her derived from her circumstances. She was one of the fortunate few for whom health costs are not a problem. She could devote her remarkable energy to her family and to others, without fear of financial ruin. This air of confidence, combined with good taste and sophistication, lent her a spirit of freshness that we seldom observed in that busy clinic.

When Mrs. Saif greeted me, I could immediately sense the bond between this strikingly lovely woman and her stunted, misshapen child. They both had broad smiles of welcome that seemed to warm the entire hallway. Dayem's father stood just behind Dayem and his mother, the two younger brothers at their father's side. He looked like the picture of a successful Middle Eastern businessman. His Savile Row blue suit fit him perfectly; his shirt and silk tie were immaculate. There was not a speck of dust on his brightly shined shoes. Mr. Saif too greeted me warmly with an Old World courtesy.

I led the family into one of our small examination rooms and then, noticing that there were not enough chairs for all of us, suggested that the younger brothers go out to the play area. They glanced at their father, whose eyes turned slightly toward the door. Without a word, the boys left the room. I lifted my tiny patient onto the examination table and stood beside him while he looked me over curiously. His smile had become a slightly mischievous grin. I felt his hand creep into mine, and I squeezed it gently. We held hands for a few moments as his parents began to tell me his medical history and that of his family. I gave Dayem a stethoscope to examine so that he wouldn't pay attention to the conversation.

Mr. Saif started by emphasizing that they had come to see me because for the past five and a half of his six years Dayem had been progressively crippled by his disease. They wanted, he said, to give their eldest son a life worth living.

Mrs. Saif provided the details of the story. Dayem's father was born in Iran, where his family has lived for more than three hundred years. Dayem's paternal great-grandfather had been a wealthy trader, first in horses and camels and later in oil. Dayem's paternal grandfather settled for a time in Syria, where his sons were the first in the family to receive formal higher education. They attended the university in Damascus. Immediately after Mr. Saif received his degree in 1951, he entered the family business and ever since has been involved in international trade, particularly petroleum product exports.

I interrupted to ask Mr. Saif whether there were known cases of thalassemia in his family. He said he knew of none. The few early deaths in his family were associated with high fever and sounded like episodes of severe infections.

Dayem's mother traced her family back to fifteenth-century Mecca. After wandering to Morocco and Egypt, they finally settled in Damascus, where she too attended the university. Mrs. Saif's great-grandfather was a governor in the Ottoman Empire, and one of his sons became a physician after attending the university in Damascus. Trained in France in lung diseases, he returned to Syria to join the Ministry of Health. His brother became an international lawyer and represented Syria at the International Court of Justice at The Hague. His sister was the second female lawyer in Damascus.

Dayem's maternal grandfather was married in Damascus and had two daughters, the younger of whom was Dayem's mother. There were no known cases of thalassemia in this branch of the family, though we later learned that Mrs. Saif's mother carried one thalassemia gene.

Mrs. Saif entered law school in Damascus, became caught up in the amalgam of socialism and nationalism that led to the short-lived United Arab Republic, and developed a political rebelliousness that she would later find necessary to repress following her marriage to her executive husband. It was obvious, however, that just beneath the surface of this refined and tactful lady lurked the young rebel of pre-Assad days. Following the death of her father and the destruction of the fledgling Syrian Republic, her mother and sister emigrated first to Beirut and then to the safety of Paris. For them, life in the Middle East was finished.

Business opportunities brought the Saifs to Lisbon in 1960, where Dayem, the first of their three sons, was born two years later. He was a small but entirely healthy and attractive-looking newborn who fed well and grew normally in the first year. In 1963, when Dayem had just turned one, a baby brother was born. At a routine visit, the family's pediatrician noted that Dayem's spleen was enlarged. He had never previously cared for Arab children and passingly wondered if the large spleen represented some sort of racial trait.

That year, Dayem caught a cold and began to look pale. The pallor persisted even after the cold symptoms abated. His rate of growth slowed, but as time went on his forehead grew large and his nose widened and flattened. The pediatrician was puzzled. When a laboratory test revealed that Dayem was anemic, his low red blood cell count was initially attributed to simple iron deficiency. After supplemental iron and vitamins did nothing to improve his red cell count, the pediatrician feared leukemia. But microscopic inspection of Dayem's red cells revealed a very different abnormality. Of the few red cells that could be counted in his blood, most were grossly misshapen and deficient in hemoglobin, the red protein that carries oxygen from the lungs to the tissues.

A normal mature red cell has no nucleus because the nucleus is shed before the fully developed cell leaves its birthplace in the bone marrow. But many of Dayem's red cells contained whole nuclei, or their remnants, indicating that they had been pushed prematurely into the blood from the bone marrow. Only a few of the red cells had a relatively normal shape and hemoglobin content, and later it was determined that these cells contained fetal hemoglobin—the type of hemoglobin that is normally present in the red cells of fetuses and infants but not in children and adults. The vast majority of Dayem's red cells were virtually useless as oxygen carriers. They contained very little adult hemoglobin and virtually no fetal hemoglobin.

In the Lisbon hospital, when Dayem's blood was spun in a centrifuge to separate the red cells from the plasma in which they were suspended, his physicians gathered further evidence of a profound defect in red cell production. His plasma was not the usual clear, straw-colored fluid. Instead, it exhibited a nasty-looking mixture of green, yellow, and brown hues. Those colors made the doctors know at once that Dayem's body must be destroying his red blood cells at a very rapid rate. When red cells are destroyed, their hemoglobin is squirted into body fluids such as plasma, where circulating chemicals change it from red to green, yellow, and brown. Given the abnormal appearance of Dayem's red blood cells, the color of his plasma, and his racial background, the pediatrician strongly suspected that Dayem was dying of thalassemia.

Though the inherited disease called thalassemia is ancient and very common on the borders of the Mediterranean Sea and in the Middle East, Far East, and Africa, the disorder was not described in the medical literature until 1924, when Dr. Thomas Cooley, a pediatrician in Detroit, Michigan, recorded five cases there. Similarly, sickle cell anemia, another ancient and common inherited disease of hemoglobin seen chiefly among black Africans, was not described until 1910 by James Herrick, a Chicago physician. It is interesting that two of the most frequent diseases in the old world were initially described in immigrants to the new world. Perhaps the physicians in southern Europe and the very few health care workers in Africa dismissed the conditions as manifestations of common infections, whereas American physicians saw them as unusual new diseases.

Red blood cells are tiny bags of a precious red protein called hemoglobin. They are pumped by the heart through mile after mile of the circulation. Like continuous commuters never allowed to leave the train, they ride in the bloodstream, their hemoglobin carrying oxygen from the lungs to the tissues until, at about one hundred days of age, they are engulfed by the spleen or liver and die. Normally the factories that produce red blood cells are located exclusively in the spongy bone marrow that occupies the hollow cavities inside the ribs, spine, hips, and pelvis. But in response to severe and sustained anemia, such as that produced by thalassemia, the red blood cell factories expand to fill every hollow space in every bone of the body, from the top of the skull to the tips of the toes. The factories even expand into the liver and spleen, which become grossly enlarged.

The red blood cell factories in bones are like automobile assembly lines. The initial product in an auto plant doesn't look much like a car at all, but as parts are added, it grows more and more familiar. Red blood cells start as big nondescript cells that have large nuclei, but before they leave the plant three changes occur: (1) the cells divide, multiply, and become smaller; (2) hemoglobin genes "turn on" to instruct the cell in the production of hemoglobin, which fills the cells; and (3) the nuclei shrink and are expelled. Once the cells are liberated into the bloodstream, their rich red hemoglobin carries oxygen throughout the body.

In the type of thalassemia from which Dayem suffered, the first and third stages of red blood cell development occur. His red blood cells divide and get smaller, and the nuclei shrink just as they should (though they are not always expelled). But a pair of very important hemoglobin genes fail to turn on. Only a paltry amount of hemoglobin is produced in each cell, and the result is a red cell without any innards. Most of these abnormal cells die before they can leave the marrow, and the few that emerge do so prematurely and are rapidly destroyed in the spleen and liver, which leads to anemia—a shortage of red blood cells in the circulation. When anemia is severe, it causes heart failure, because the muscles and electrical system of the heart are deprived of adequate oxygen.

But bodies, like prizefighters, usually don't go down with the first punch. In response to the anemia, the marrow assembly line frantically increases its effort to produce red blood cells. The head and face become distorted as the bones of the skull take up the task of red cell production. The bones of the arms, legs, ribs, back, and hips are weakened by the huge expansion of their marrow cores. The liver and spleen grow so large that they compress the stomach and intestines. Growth of the body is terribly retarded because the long bones do not develop properly, and fractures are common—all of this in response to two defective hemoglobin genes.

Dayem and all human beings have several different pairs of hemoglobin genes. One member of each pair is inherited from the father, and the other member of the pair is inherited from the mother. It happened that Dayem's father and his mother both carried one normal and one defective member of a pair of particularly important hemoglobin genes, called beta globin genes. Dayem's misfortune was that each parent passed their defective gene on to their son, leaving him no normal beta globin gene with which to make hemoglobin. This deficiency crippled his red cell assembly line and caused his red cells to die aborning.

Such is the roulette of genetics. Dayem might have drawn a normal gene from each parent, as did one of his brothers. If he had done so, he would have been entirely healthy. He might have drawn one abnormal gene from one parent and one normal gene from the other parent, as did his other brother, and if he had done so, he would have been no worse off than either of his parents, who each have only one good beta globin gene. But Dayem was unlucky; he drew two defective genes.

When the Lisbon pediatrician tentatively diagnosed thalassemia, a disorder Dayem's parents had no idea they were carrying, the parents requested a second opinion. They were referred to the foremost pediatric hematologist in Europe, Guido Fanconi of the Kinderspital in Zurich. Fanconi, a stately gentleman then in his seventies, sadly confirmed the Lisbon opinion. Dayem had severe thalassemia, an ultimately fatal inherited disease for which the only known treatment was repeated transfusion of red cells, a therapy which Fanconi emphasized is itself eventually fatal.

The late Guido Fanconi was a well-established consultant. He and his younger associate, Walter Hitzig, were among the most experienced pediatric hematologists in Europe, and often they had had to give grim news to parents from around the world. Fanconi spoke frankly and carefully, but his message was chillingly clear. Dayem would die of anemia unless he received regular transfusions, but if he did receive transfusions, he would die during his teen years or before because the iron that is present in the transfused red cells would accumulate and overload the body. Either anemia or iron overload would eventually kill him. It might be better to withhold transfusions—let Dayem live his short life and die in peace.

But Fanconi offered one faint hope. Thalassemia, even in its severe form, is a very unpredictable disease, in part because the defects in hemoglobin genes are variable among the nationalities in which the genetic abnormalities have arisen. One or both of the thalassemia mutations that Dayem had inherited might be a relatively milder type. Therefore, it was barely possible that his circulating red cells and the precious hemoglobin they contained might be sufficient to sustain his life without lethal blood transfusions.

Fanconi had little experience of patients from Syria and Iran, and could say no more about this remote possibility. Yet it was Dayem's only hope for survival into young adult life.

"Have no more children," Fanconi cautioned the Saifs, who at this point had only one other son. "You have a 25 percent chance of bearing a thalassemic child with each pregnancy."

Mrs. Saif had listened fixedly to every word. She had given up a professional career when she married, and now, she realized, her career would be the life of her first-born child. She and her husband would care for Dayem without transfusions and pray that his enfeebled red cell production would be sufficient to sustain him. They would not support him temporarily with transfusions only to lose him in a few years as a result of the treatment itself. With sorrow and determination, they returned to Lisbon, their lives irrevocably changed. They would continue to conduct their business and social affairs as they had always done, but they would forever bear the burden of guilt that plagues the parents of children with severe inherited diseases.

Dayem was then less than two years old. What, they wondered, would be his feelings about them when he grew older? Would he hate them for what they had done to him? They had each harbored a bad seed. Its presence had been utterly unknown to them, but each of these seeds had been revealed in its ugly form because, by chance, both had been deposited in their innocent son. Was this a cruel twist of fate from which all of them would suffer, or would this be a test that would determine whether they had the power to snatch something of value from an apparent disaster?

Dayem did not, after all, receive his defective hemoglobin genes only from them. The genes had passed through them from the generations that had preceded, and they would continue to be passed to successive generations. To be guilty of passing thalassemia was to be guilty of no more than being a Syrian, an Iranian, or one of a vast number of ancestral groups in which the thalassemia genes are common. No, they decided, they would not gaze guiltily or shamefully at their first-born son. The test before them was to give him a worthwhile life. When they returned to Lisbon, the battle for Dayem's life began.

FOR A TIME, Dayem did reasonably well without transfusion, but one day when he was three years old and his brother was two, both boys were invited to a birthday party. They sat in the back of the family limousine, without seat belts, on their way to the party when suddenly the driver stopped to avoid an accident. Dayem fell to the floor and developed severe pain in his lower leg. The leg appeared a bit swollen. An x-ray showed a fracture of the tibia—the first incident in what his mother calls his fracture period. During that year Dayem fractured his left arm and his other tibia. He even fractured a finger without knowing it. Then when Dayem was four, his family traveled to Cascais, a summer resort in Portugal. As his grandmother took Dayem by the hand to show him to his bedroom, he separated from her, slipped on the parquet floor, and broke his femur, the large bone in his thigh. He remained in a body cast for two months.

Between the ages of four and six, every picture of Dayem in the family album shows him with a cast; the cast became part and parcel of him. It was impossible to send him to school. A teacher came to the house, but she was much too slow for this bright boy. He disliked her tremendously.

From the time the fracture period began to the time I first saw him in the autumn of 1968, Dayem had broken almost every bone in his body. He had gotten out of an arm cast only a few days before he came to Boston. If this was the true meaning of the "peaceful" life and death Dr. Fanconi offered, the Saifs concluded that there had to be another way.

When Dayem was three and a half years old, and in the midst of the fracture episodes, his mother became pregnant again. This time she was badly frightened. Fanconi's advice rang in her ears, and she strongly considered an abortion. Her husband was against the idea but left the final decision to her. She decided to have the baby, and the third son was born. She watched him constantly for pallor and felt his belly every day to see whether his spleen or liver was enlarging. To her immense joy and relief, he proved, after a year, to be entirely normal.

By early 1968, Dayem's pediatricians also began to wonder whether his lack of treatment was truly appropriate. Having learned of my research on thalassemia, they suggested that his parents bring him to see me at Children's Hospital in Boston.

On their way to Boston from Lisbon, the Saifs had taken a detour, first to Beirut and then to Paris, for a long family vacation. It would be their last for some time; once they arrived in America, Mr. Saif plunged into responsibility for his company's interests in all of Latin America.

Dayem was so pale when I first saw him, and his heart was pumping so rapidly, that I found it difficult to believe he could have traveled anywhere. But the Saifs insisted that the vacation had been delightful. Family and friends were awed by Dayem's quick mind and sociability, despite his physical impairments. His bones had remained intact throughout the trip, and he had particularly enjoyed Beirut. Sadly, because of the worsening political situation there, it was the last trip to Beirut for him or for anyone else in the family. Shortly thereafter, that once-beautiful city, hailed as the Paris of the Middle East, became chaotic and dangerous.

The family had traveled from France to New York on the last great French oceanliner, *The France*. Dayem, though very pale and frail, had been full of life, taking good care of his brothers and remaining the leader of the trio despite his small size. When every member of the family except Dayem became seasick, he kept up their spirits during five rather miserable, stormy days. He and his brothers covered every inch of the rocking ship, climbing over forbidden guard rails, hiding under lifeboats, and playing in the elevators. On one particularly stormy afternoon, the seasick parents lay groaning in their cabin and finally fell asleep. When they awakened with a start near dinner time, there was no sign of their boys. They dashed up onto the upper decks, enlisting the aid of stewards to find them. Waves were crashing against the bow, the ship creaked and rocked. They forgot their nausea as fear replaced it.

Suddenly, staggering against the wind and spray, Dayem appeared around the corner of the radio shack, holding the hands of his shivering brothers. "They got cold and wet," he explained. "I thought I should bring them in." The parents looked at each other incredulously. "Yes," said Mr. Saif. "Let's go in."

I was astonished to hear of Dayem's playfulness and sense of responsibility for his brothers on board, because by the time I examined him in Boston he was so terribly pale. In fact, his hemoglobin was the lowest value that we have ever recorded in a patient who walked into the clinic on his own, 1.5 grams per hundred milliliters of blood! Normal hemoglobin for a boy his age is at least 10.5 grams per hundred milliliters. (One gram is about 3/100 of a solid ounce, and one milliliter is about 3/100 of a liquid ounce.) Dayem's hemoglobin concentration was only ten percent of normal. How he could have played in that cold, rocking ship remains a mystery—one of many.

As soon as they received Dayem's blood sample, the laboratory technicians called me in alarm. They wanted to be sure I knew how low his red cell count was. When they rapidly analyzed the components of his hemoglobin, they found that about half of the residual protein was normal adult hemoglobin (hemoglobin A) and half was fetal hemoglobin (hemoglobin F)—the type of hemoglobin that is found in all fetal red cells. Patients with severe thalassemia, whose pair of defective beta globin genes cannot produce adequate adult hemoglobin, may still be able to produce variable amounts of fetal hemoglobin, because another pair of hemoglobin genes—called gamma—"turn on." Dayem produced a few red blood cells that contained fetal hemoglobin, and they tended to survive because they were better filled.

Because some of the hemoglobin in Dayem's blood was the normal adult type, Dr. Fanconi's hope had been at least partially realized. Dayem did not have the most severe type of thalassemia. At least one or both of his thalassemic beta globin genes were capable of making a very small amount of normal adult hemoglobin. But the amount was much too small to fill his red blood cells. Hence his severe marrow disease and liver and spleen enlargement—all due to the premature death of his developing red blood cells and the constant production of more defective, useless cells to replace them.

Most of the few circulating red blood cells Dayem did have were very bizarre. Instead of the well-filled and evenly shaped red cells of normal individuals, Dayem had some that were tiny fragments, some that looked like pale empty platters, and others that resem-

bled teardrops. The only cells that seemed well filled with hemoglobin and had a normal shape (perhaps 10 or 20 percent of
Dayem's few cells) were those that contained relatively large
amounts of fetal hemoglobin (figure 1).

While the laboratory was studying Dayem's blood on that first
day in our clinic, he lay rather comfortably on the examination
table, but his breathing could be heard down the hallway. His
pulse was rapid and his chest heaved with every heartbeat. Though
he had walked into the clinic, I became very concerned that he
would go into severe heart failure before my eyes. I gingerly lifted
him into a wheelchair and admitted him to the hospital for his
first blood transfusion.

When I announced that Dayem must be treated with red cell
transfusions, his mother immediately reminded me of Dr. Fanconi's
warning. I agreed that there were serious risks, but I thought we had
to take them. We needed to correct Dayem's severe anemia and
thereby protect his heart from imminent failure. And we also
needed to give transfusions to protect his bones, by shutting off
secretion of the hormone that induces red blood cell formation.

That hormone is made in the kidneys and travels in the blood
to the bone marrow, where it stimulates red cell production. The

Normal and Thalassemia Red Cells

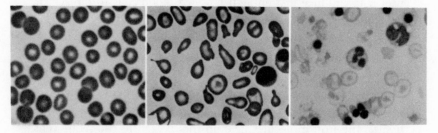

Figure 1 Normal red blood cells are concave disks of similar diameter
that are well filled with hemoglobin (left photomicrograph). By contrast,
Dayem's red cells had many different shapes, and some were nucleated
(middle). After his spleen was removed, most of his red cells looked like
targets (right), with only a central "bull's eye" of hemoglobin. Most were
nucleated and pale; the few red cells that were well filled contained quite
a bit of fetal hemoglobin.

kidneys of patients with any severe anemia, including thalassemia, produce excessive amounts of the hormone, which obediently circulates to the marrow and stimulates more and more red cell production. Unfortunately, in the case of thalassemia, these newly formed red blood cells are defective and therefore are immediately swallowed by the rubbish-eating cells that reside in the marrow, spleen, and liver. The patient remains anemic, and therefore more and more red-cell-production hormone is manufactured. The bony walls of the marrow spaces expand to keep up with the demand, the bones weaken, and multiple fractures and stunted growth are the result. The body gets drawn into a vicious downward spiral of failure, overcompensation, and destruction.

If the excessive birth of red blood cells and the huge expansion of the bony walls of the marrow spaces are to be reduced, the hormone production must be suppressed. Transfusion is a bypass mechanism which, by correcting anemia, shuts off the hormone. Therefore, I treated all of our thalassemia patients with a high red cell transfusion program that would ensure that their bones would be permitted to thicken.

Lethal iron overload is the inevitable consequence of regular and repeated red cell transfusion in nonbleeding patients. In normal people, about one percent of the circulating red blood cells die every day. The iron they contain is recycled to the marrow, which uses it to produce just enough new red blood cells to replace the dead ones. Iron is therefore retained in the red cells, and very little spills over into the tissues.

Iron plays a particularly vital role in the function of hemoglobin. When a red cell that is devoid of oxygen is pumped by the heart to the lungs, the iron molecules in the hemoglobin each grab a molecule of oxygen. When the red cell is pumped to the tissues, the iron molecules give up the oxygen to the tissue cells. Within the tissue cells, the oxygen is immediately put to work to burn food.

Much of this combustion is accomplished by the microscopic furnaces of the cell. These organelles convert sugar, fat, and amino acids (protein) into stored energy and heat. They accomplish this conversion by using certain other proteins that also require iron for their normal function. Thus, the tiny amount of iron that finds its way into cells other than red cells is used to govern oxygen movement by the microscopic energy furnaces that exist in nearly all of the cells of the body. Absent iron, the furnaces won't work and the cells die.

Chronic red cell transfusion completely disrupts normal iron metabolism. The entire content of iron in a child of six is no more than 1.5 grams. But every milliliter of red cells contains a milligram of iron (1/1000 of a gram). If we give a six-year-old child two pints of red cells every six weeks to increase his circulating hemoglobin, we will have given this child almost five grams of iron per year. This is more than four times the child's total body iron content. Furthermore, the child can't get rid of the iron from the tissues unless he or she bleeds or makes more red blood cells, and this defeats the transfusion's purpose entirely.

So the child continues to accumulate iron in the tissues up to the point at which it begins to do much more harm than good. After a few years, the huge mass of iron begins to act like an electric wire. A flow of electricity moves through the expanded iron pools and begins to "electrocute" the tissues very slowly but steadily. The liver, the pancreas, and particularly the heart are very vulnerable to such "electrocution." When heart cells are finally damaged beyond repair, the child slowly dies of heart failure.

That was my dilemma when I first saw Dayem. It was a dilemma I faced in all of my patients with thalassemia. Somehow I would have to solve it.

While we waited for the blood to come from the transfusion service, the Saifs continued to press me about the long-term consequences of transfusion therapy. They were particularly concerned about the iron in the blood, but they had also heard of other complications of transfusion and wanted to be reassured that the risks would be minimized.

I had to agree that transfusion carries a risk of infection such as hepatitis in addition to iron overload, but the risk was low in our experience. Our transfusion service was highly trained and our blood was obtained from carefully screened donors who were largely family members and friends of our patients and staff. The danger of hepatitis carried by our donors was very small, though not nonexistent. Transfusion-induced AIDS was not known at the time.

I explained the facts as I knew them to the Saifs in simple terms, but I noticed that they asked for details and were particularly concerned about Dayem's schedule of transfusions. They wanted to know why the transfusions couldn't be spaced far enough apart to lessen the accumulation of iron, even if Dayem remained mildly anemic. They knew that mild anemia would not put Dayem at risk for heart failure, and they worried that iron overload would make heart failure a certainty.

I reemphasized that patients with thalassemia must receive enough red cells to maintain a near-normal hemoglobin level until the next transfusion, in order to suppress red-cell-production hormone. Since the red cells in a unit of blood live an average of sixty days, we usually transfuse patients at about monthly intervals, to ensure that the patient's hemoglobin level will not drop below the threshold at which red-cell-production hormone is secreted. I recognized that this schedule would produce iron overload, but no other approach would save Dayem's bones from fracture and permit him to grow. I admitted that the iron overload would be lethal eventually unless research turned up some way to get the excess iron out of his body, but he would die immediately if we failed to act now. They understood and reluctantly assented to the long-term transfusion program.

At the end of this first meeting with the Saifs, I told them that I would do my best to find a way out of the dilemma that faced Dayem and all of the patients like him. They looked at each other, then Mr. Saif spoke. "We do trust you, doctor. We've come this far to see you because we are told that you will try. So will we."

THE INTERNS, residents, and students on the ward were as taken aback as I when they saw Dayem for the first time. His hemoglobin was so low and his heart so close to failure that they simply could not believe that he had been wandering around the outside world and had even just completed a transatlantic voyage. "This boy must have nine lives," one of them offered.

It was a prophetic comment, but not as interesting as the words of a young Lebanese who had just come to Children's Hospital as a fellow in immunology. He happened to be on the ward when Dayem was admitted.

"My God, what's that?" he whispered to me.

"It's my patient—Dayem Saif," I answered with a note of irritation and pride.

"I can't believe he's alive. His name must be making him immortal."

"What do you mean—what about his name?"

"Oh, of course, you don't know Arabic. Dayem Saif means 'immortal sword.'"

I went over to the bed, looked again at the tiny fellow and thought to myself, "Well, my little Immortal Sword—we've got a long battle to fight together. You better live up to that name."

Killer or Savior

DAYEM'S first transfusion took us two long days. We transfused slowly so that his heart would have plenty of time to adjust to the new load. Thankfully, Dayem did not go into heart failure. In fact, he became the hit of the ward. The staff saw his courage and humor more than his tiny frail body and distorted face.

While the first transfusion was being slowly administered, the Saifs and I had plenty of opportunity to talk about thalassemia. Their overwhelming feeling was guilt. How, they kept asking, had they done this to their son? I could help them very little with their sorrow, but I could give them the facts as I saw them.

"Blame it all on malaria," I insisted. "Thalassemia has nothing to do with what you and your families did. It has everything to do with the Anopheles mosquito." If the malaria parasite (a protozoan) and its insect partner, the Anopheles mosquito, had not been widespread in parts of the Middle East, Africa, and Asia, thalassemia would scarcely exist because the thalassemia mutation is not a favorable one—by itself it impedes survival and reproduction. However, the thalassemia gene has one good thing going for it: to some degree, it protects those who carry it against death from malaria, and in populations where malaria is a threat, this protection outweighs the threat of thalassemia posed by the defective gene itself. In evolutionary terms, we might say that thalassemia genes have offered more benefit than risk overall in environments where malaria occurs. That's why the gene has survived.

Genetic mutations are random changes that occur very rarely in some genes and with higher frequency in others. Mutations in the hemoglobin genes occur relatively frequently, but they usually do not persist or concentrate in one ethnic population unless there is a significant amount of intermarriage. The reason a defective gene such as thalassemia would ordinarily fade out is this: though "thalassemia trait" (meaning one thalassemia gene and one normal gene) is innocuous, severe thalassemia (two thalassemia genes) is fatal long before its victims are old enough to have children of their own. Therefore, couples carrying this deleterious gene are at a reproductive disadvantage: on average, fewer of their offspring would survive and have children of their own than would be the case among normal couples. However, in the old malarious world such as the Mediterranean basin, the defective gene has persisted because a form of malaria (called falciparum malaria) kills children who have two *normal* hemoglobin genes more effectively than it kills those with one thalassemia gene and one normal gene. As a result, the prevalence of the different genes for thalassemia has steadily increased in those regions where malaria is a danger.

When a man and a woman who each have thalassemia trait, like Mr. and Mrs. Saif, have children, there is a 25 percent chance of having a baby like Dayem with two thalassemia genes and severe disease. Children with two thalassemia genes die before they can have babies of their own, and therefore do not contribute to the "gene pool" of the next generation. But their failure to have children does not affect the upward march of the thalassemia gene in the community, because falciparum malaria slows down the survival and reproductive rate of "normals" to a greater extent than thalassemia slows down those rates among people who bear one thalassemia gene. By the time the population has figured out how to reduce the incidence of malaria by attacking the parasite or the mosquito, the frequency of the thalassemia gene has reached very high proportions.

Common sense would dictate that at this point the birthrate of children severely ill with thalassemia would also increase. And since severe thalassemics die before they have children, the number of thalassemia genes in the community would begin to decline.

That is in fact what happens: eventually, the number of individuals who have two normal hemoglobin genes becomes balanced by those who have one abnormal thalassemia gene and one normal gene. This state of affairs is known as "balanced polymorphism," a term that describes the fact that a gene like thalassemia, which protects from malaria, will increase its frequency until its prevalence in the population is balanced by the failure of those who are severely affected to have children and spread the gene.

We do not know precisely how thalassemia genes provide protection from lethal falciparum malaria. Recent work suggests that when thalassemia-trait red cells become infected by falciparum malaria parasites, they are more effectively destroyed by the immune system than are infected normal red cells, but this may not be the only mechanism. Whatever the cause, it is extraordinary to see how effective thalassemia trait has been in increasing the survival advantage of individuals who carry it. A few spontaneous thalassemia mutations which occurred probably thousands of years ago in the eggs or sperm of a handful of individuals living in highly malarious regions expanded so much in the population that, today, a very high percentage of people in many parts of the world have become carriers of the gene. A map of the world distribution of beta thalassemia reflects the accumulation of this mutant gene, under environmental pressure from malaria (figure 2).

The spread of the thalassemia gene (before the advent of modern techniques to combat malaria) is in many ways a beautiful if tragic confirmation of Charles Darwin's principle of evolution through natural selection. The environment produced "selection pressure" in the form of malaria. A trait which, in a different environment, would have been evolutionarily disadvantageous (because those carrying it would be unable to reproduce as successfully as normal individuals) became evolutionarily advantageous when reproduction among normal individuals fell off as a result of malaria. "Fitness" for survival, as Darwin knew very well, is clearly a relative concept: it depends on the nature of the environment at any given time and, equally important, on the strength of the local competition.

The prevalence of the beta thalassemia gene has become enormous in some areas of the world. In parts of Italy and Greece, as many as 15 percent of the population had beta thalassemia trait in 1961 (the year of the most recent survey that I could report to the Saifs). There were approximately two million Italians with thalassemia trait, and each year approximately one thousand children were born who inherited two defective genes and therefore had severe disease. The prevalence of the thalassemia gene was 10 percent in the valley of the Po River, in Sicily, and in Calabria, Lucania, Puglia, and Campania. In southern Sardinia, it was as high as 30 percent. The average prevalence in Greece was 7 percent, rising to as high as 10 percent in the Arta district and in northern and central Greece. As a result, the frequency of new cases of severe thalassemia approached two hundred per year in that country.

The frequency of the gene was 10 percent on most of the Aegean islands, up to 25 percent in Rhodes, and 15 percent in

The World Distribution of Beta Thalassemia

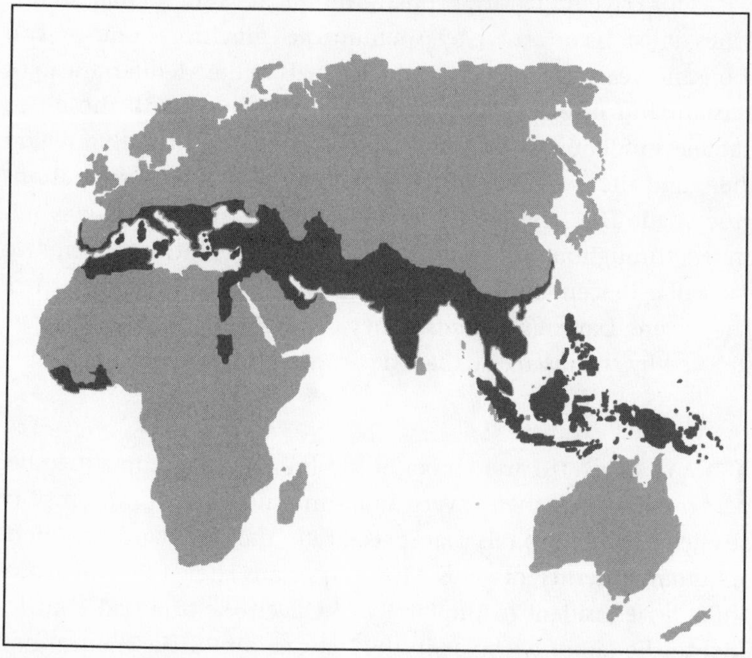

Figure 2 The dark shaded areas show regions of the world where frequencies of falciparum malaria, and therefore beta thalassemia, are high.

Cyprus. It was common in Bulgaria, Turkey, Israel, Syria, Iran, southern Russia, and particularly in the Persian Gulf littoral. In Israel, the incidence was very high among Kurdish Jews, but it was almost never seen in Ashkenazi Jews, providing further evidence of the different genealogic histories of these two populations. India had a highly variable incidence of beta thalassemia trait. In some of the communities in Bangladesh, the rate was nearly 15 percent, and was as high as 8 percent in the Sindhi population near Bombay. In Thailand the frequency ranged from 4 percent to 10 percent, and it was high in Malaysian and Indonesian populations as well. The incidence of the gene was extremely variable in Africa; the highest frequency was found in the areas of West Africa where there is a lot of malaria. Given these tremendously high incidences of thalassemia trait in much of the world, it was estimated that somewhere between 100,000 and 300,000 infants with severe thalassemia were born each year. Most died in the first twelve months of life.

As for Dayem's family, I concluded that at least two thalassemia genes must have arisen by spontaneous mutations one or two thousand years ago in different individuals in the Mediterranean or Persian Gulf littoral of the Middle East. We might call those two nameless individuals founders. Malaria was rampant in that region then, and the frequency of the genes increased as the generations proceeded. The descendants of those who carried the genes migrated throughout the Arab world. Many generations later, two particular descendants of the original founders met and married. They were Dayem's parents. They, and many like them, were shocked by the discovery that they carried thalassemia.

DAYEM AND I were brought together because I am a member of what was then a very small international community of physicians and hospitals that specialize in the study and treatment of human inherited diseases. Most physicians knew that the hemophilia gene resident in the family of Queen Victoria had contributed to the fall of Nicholas II, the last Czar of Russia; his son had episodic joint bleeding, the pain of which responded only to hypnotic spells induced by the monk Rasputin. A few doctors were even aware that Frederick the Great of Prussia had been physically abused by his father, Frederick Wilhelm, while the latter was possessed by the explosive rages that can characterize acute intermittent porphyria, a very rare inherited defect in the synthesis of heme, the iron-containing part of hemoglobin. In general, however, there was little awareness within most health care systems of the impending scientific explosion in genetics and its implications for understanding inherited diseases, nor was there a broad commitment to the discovery of new methods of treatment.

To be sure, most high school and college students who had even the most rudimentary education in biology knew something about the contributions of Gregor Mendel (1822–1884). Mendel had created entirely new concepts of inheritance through his experiments showing that different characteristics of garden peas are passed from generation to generation in a predictable fashion. He recognized not just that different genes control different aspects of appearance but that the presence of some genes is hidden from view. Such invisible or *recessive* genes do not influence the characteristics of peas if they are present only as a single copy. These genes may, however, be passed along to the next generation. And if those second-generation peas inherit two identical recessive genes from each parent, their appearance will be affected. (In that case, we would say that these recessive genes are "expressed.") Other genes, as Mendel showed, can affect appearance (be expressed) even if they are present as a single copy. These are called *dominant* genes, and they influence appearance in every subsequent generation.

Nearly all of the students with whom I entered Harvard Medical School in 1951 had a general knowledge of the genetic rules that govern the behavior of Mendel's peas. We knew that genes are the units of heredity, and that in humans they are distributed on 46 chromosomes, two of which are the sex chromosomes, called X and Y. The remaining 44 chromosomes represent 22 pairs, each pair identifiable in the microscope by its own characteristic size and shape. Later we learned that most of the hemoglobin genes are found on the pair of chromosomes designated number 11. The rest are found on the chromosomes designated 16. Since embryos receive one chromosome 11 and one chromosome 16 from the sperm or the egg of each parent, we must inherit half of our hemoglobin genes—indeed half of all of our genes—from each parent.

We knew from the work of Oswald Avery and his colleagues at Rockefeller University carried out in the 1940s that genes are made of DNA. Not long thereafter, Erwin Chargaff at Columbia University had demonstrated that DNA is made up of four smaller molecules, called nucleotides, that are linked together by sugar and phosphate molecules into a huge chain of DNA. The nucleotides of DNA—adenine (A), guanine (G), thymine (T), and cytosine (C)—are the code words in the genes that regulate all of life and are passed to subsequent generations on the chromosomes.

Later we would learn how this genetic code is read in the cell so that proteins are produced. But before we could be concerned about the precise nature of the code, we had to understand how the code words themselves are passed to subsequent generations, that is, how the chromosomes and the DNA replicate. These questions were answered in part in my second year of medical school when James Watson, then a postdoctoral fellow from Harvard and subsequently a Harvard professor and chairman, and Francis Crick of Cambridge University electrified the world with their discovery that DNA takes the shape of a double helix. Watson and Crick shared the 1962 Nobel Prize for physiology and medicine. Later, Watson became the director of the Cold Spring Harbor Laboratory, where many important discoveries in genetics were made.

The two strands of DNA are wound around each other like two pieces of spaghetti (figure 3). Because of the nature of their chemical bonds, the A's are always opposite T's, and the G's are always opposite C's. During replication, the strands unwind. With the assistance of specialized proteins called polymerases, each single strand is then copied. The two old strands each function as a template for a new complementary strand until all the bases are paired again, and two new double helixes are formed.

Though we medical students were struggling to understand a vast amount of science all at once, even we could grasp the enormous meaning of Watson and Crick's model. It provided a molecular explanation for DNA replication—that is, for the secret of how living cells reproduce themselves. This "unzipping" of the DNA molecule in the cell's nucleus, and the subsequent replication of the two sides of the "zipper," was the mechanism through which a parent cell passed genetic information on to its two daughter cells.

During our first two years of medical school we were regularly reminded of the emerging role genes were beginning to play in our understanding of health and disease. A major concept had come from Archibald Garrod (1857–1936), an English physician who in 1908 had described patients with a very rare inherited tendency to excrete black urine—a disorder called alkaptonuria. He proposed that patients with alkaptonuria and other inborn errors of metabolism had inherited a deficiency of specific enzymes that are vital constituents in the metabolism of particular fuels, be they sugars, fats, or the amino acids derived from proteins. Enzymes are proteins that act as catalysts, speeding the rate at which a biochemical reaction proceeds but not altering the nature of the reaction. When an enzyme deficiency occurs, metabolism of sugar, fat, or amino acid slows down or is interrupted altogether; in other words, the

The Replication of DNA

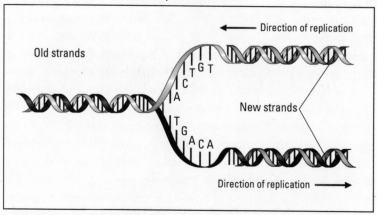

Figure 3 DNA is made of two strands of nucleotides that wind around each other to form a double helix. The strands are held together by weak bonds between individual nucleotides, where an A in one strand is always opposite a T in the other, and a G is always opposite a C. During replication, the coils separate, and each coil forms a template for the synthesis of a new molecule of DNA. Replication proceeds in opposite directions.

enzyme deficiency creates a roadblock in a metabolic pathway. In the case of alkaptonuria, a black-colored product of incomplete amino acid breakdown accumulates at the roadblock and is excreted in the urine.

Four decades later, another important concept came from two American geneticists at Stanford University, George Beadle and Edward Tatum. They examined the metabolic behavior of a certain bread mold and correctly proposed that *all* metabolic pathways are controlled by enzymes, which are themselves produced by genes. A block in a metabolic reaction is likely to be caused by a defective or absent enzyme, and the enzyme failure is likely to be caused by a defective or absent gene. These proposals—so simple and straightforward in hindsight—set the stage for understanding all of medical genetics; and in recognition of their important contributions, Beadle and Tatum were awarded the Nobel Prize for physiology and medicine in 1958.

As for my own area of special interest—inherited abnormalities in hemoglobin—important milestones in our understanding of that molecule's structure were established in the 1940s while I was still in high school poring over diagrams of hybrid crosses in Mendel's peas. At that time James Neel, a third-year medical student at Rochester University School of Medicine, and William Valentine, then a medical resident at Rochester, joined forces to study Italian-American families in which at least one family member had severe thalassemia. Both of them had become fascinated by a patient they had seen, and both had read Maxwell Wintrobe's famous textbook of hematology to learn more about it. Wintrobe had described a mild form of thalassemia, and what interested Neel and Valentine was the genetics of severe thalassemia. Would both parents and some siblings of those with severe disease have the mild form of the disease and have only one defective hemoglobin gene, they wondered, while those with severe disease would have two—one inherited from each parent? Their studies of the Italian-American population of Rochester established that vital point.

Meanwhile, in 1945 William B. Castle, a professor of medicine at Harvard Medical School, and Linus Pauling, a Nobel-Prize-winning biophysicist at the California Institute of Technology, found themselves together on an overnight train from Denver to Chicago. To pass the time, Castle began to tell Pauling what he knew about sickle cell anemia. Sickle red cells, he explained, owe their peculiar sickle shape not to some intrinsic deformity of the red cell membrane but to a strong tendency of sickle cell hemoglobin itself to elongate into rod-like forms when it is depleted of oxygen. The rods of hemoglobin distort the red cell and create the sickle cell deformity which in turn causes all of the symptoms of sickle cell disease, including episodes of severe bone pain, death of cells in the liver and brain, and bouts of pneumonia. Castle convinced Pauling that a mutation of a hemoglobin gene must be responsible for these rod-like forms and hoped that Pauling would work on the problem.

When Pauling returned to California, he instructed his student, Harvey Itano, to find a way to separate sickle from normal protein. In 1949 Pauling and Itano published the now-classical experiment demonstrating that sickle hemoglobin could be separated from normal hemoglobin in an electrical field. Patients with sickle cell anemia had almost 100 percent sickle hemoglobin in their red cells and no normal adult hemoglobin, while individuals with sickle trait but no symptoms of disease had both sickle and normal adult hemoglobins in their cells.

This observation confirmed and extended another of James Neel's investigations. He had become a faculty member at the University of Michigan and had studied patients with sickle cell anemia and their parents in Detroit. He concluded that both parents of these patients had sickle trait, just as he had earlier demonstrated that both parents of children with severe thalassemia had thalassemia trait.

Hemoglobin—or any protein—represents a long chain of well over one hundred much smaller molecules called amino acids (figure 4). There are only twenty different amino acids in living organisms. All the different proteins in the human body, from insulin to hemoglobin to heart muscle, are made up of some combination and repetition of these twenty building blocks.

Pauling and Itano concluded that sickle hemoglobin must be due to an amino acid substitution, in which one "correct" amino

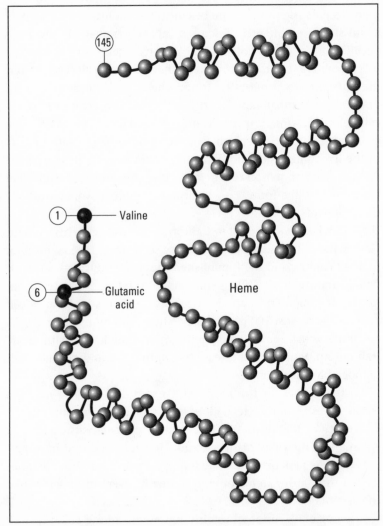

Figure 4 The human beta globin chain contains 145 amino acids, beginning with valine. The particular sequence of amino acids causes the protein to fold in a unique fashion, forming a large pocket in which a molecule of heme that carries oxygen can fit. One amino acid can usually be substituted for another without any change in the shape of the molecule, but if the glutamic acid at position 6 is replaced by a valine, the substitution causes sickle cell anemia. Many other such "point mutations" can cause different types of thalassemia.

acid is replaced by another "incorrect" one. And such a change, they argued, must be governed by a mutation in a hemoglobin gene. The precise amino acid substitution that produces sickle hemoglobin rather than normal adult hemoglobin was reported ten years later by Vernon Ingram, then in England and now a professor at the Massachusetts Institute of Technology.

The proposals of Garrod and the experiments of Beadle and Tatum and Neel made clear to my medical school classmates and me that severe thalassemia and sickle cell anemia are both due to the inheritance of two defective recessive hemoglobin genes, one from each parent. Each of the parents of a patient with a severe thalassemia similar to Dayem's has barely detectable anemia, but when one examines their red cells under a microscope, they appear abnormally small. Unlike individuals with sickle cell trait, people with thalassemia trait have no abnormally shaped hemoglobin molecules in their red cells. Therefore different mutations of the hemoglobin genes that were unknown at the time must be responsible for thalassemia and sickle cell anemia respectively. Furthermore, thalassemia must be due to abnormally low production of *normal* hemoglobin rather than *normal* production of *abnormal* hemoglobin, as is the case in sickle cell anemia. If thalassemia was to be understood and treated, physicians would have to know much more about hemoglobin and the genes that govern its production.

In 1954, while I was a fourth-year medical student, Vernon Ingram proposed that hemoglobin is not a single chain of amino acids. Instead, he said, it is comprised of two different pairs of protein chains called globins. Shortly thereafter the proposal was confirmed by several groups of protein chemists. The two different globin chains are known as the alpha and beta chains. The chemical symbol for adult hemoglobin is therefore $\alpha_2\beta_2$ (figure 5).

Each globin chain has a molecule called heme attached to it which contains the iron atom that binds oxygen in the lungs and gives it up to tissues. The alpha chains are produced by alpha genes on chromosome 16, and the beta chains are produced by beta genes on chromosome 11. This discovery opened up a new approach to hemoglobin chemistry and genetics. It soon became possible to determine the exact amino acid sequence of each of the globin chains and thereafter to define precisely the amino acid substitutions that cause the inherited disorders of hemoglobin.

WHY IS HUMAN hemoglobin so complicated? Why are there two pairs of chains made by two different genes located on two different chromosomes? The answers to those questions—like so many "why?" questions—are enshrouded in the mists of evolution. We do know that more than half a billion years

Structure of Human Hemoglobin

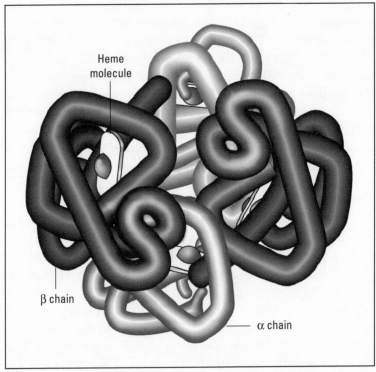

Figure 5 The adult hemoglobin molecule is made up of two alpha chains and two beta chains. The four heme molecules carrying oxygen are inserted into a pocket in each chain.

ago, the marine ancestors from which we and all other mammals eventually evolved had a single hemoglobin gene. Humans and many other higher organisms still have a rudiment of that gene. It makes the protein called myoglobin that contributes the red color to our muscles and is responsible for the rapid movement of oxygen in muscle. About 450 million years ago, for reasons that we may never understand, that single gene duplicated and split up. The myoglobin gene went off to appear later on human chromosome 22. The alpha and beta genes stayed together on one chromosome in frogs and then were passed around until, in humans, the alphas came to rest on chromosome 16 and the betas on chromosome 11.

Much more recently (between 200 and 300 million years ago) the alpha and beta genes duplicated and produced hemoglobin genes that function only in the embryo. We call these epsilon and zeta genes. They are respectively near the beta gene on chromosome 11 and the alpha genes on chromosome 16. In the process the alpha genes themselves duplicated and left two nearly identical alpha genes on chromosome 16.

About 100 million years ago, the beta gene duplicated again and formed another gene called gamma that also remained close by on chromosome 11. Fifty to seventy-five million years later, that gamma gene duplicated again, and so did the beta gene—to form a gene called delta (see figure 11 on page 177).

Therefore that cluster of beta-like genes on chromosome 11 is a busy and crowded place from conception to birth. There are five hemoglobin genes that operate there in sequence: the embryonic gene called epsilon is expressed for a few weeks after conception; then the two gamma genes operate during the rest of fetal life; following birth, the delta gene functions at a very low rate, but the beta gene turns on full force (figure 6).

Things are simpler over on chromosome 16. There the zeta gene turns on to produce a partner for the epsilon chain during the first few weeks of embryonic life. Then the two alpha genes take over and remain on, providing alpha chain partners for the products of the gamma, delta, and beta genes on chromosome 11.

There is a simple chemical explanation for all of this complex effort—and for the endurance of each of these changes throughout millions of years of evolution. Hemoglobin works much better when it is made of two different chains. It is more soluble, and it binds oxygen in the lungs and gives it up to the tissues much more effectively in this form. In fact, a hemoglobin molecule that is made of four beta chains or four gamma chains is not very soluble and gives up oxygen to tissues very poorly. On the other hand, free alpha chains—chains with no partners—are so insoluble that they can't combine or function at all. That last point turned out to be very important to Dayem, as we will see.

The fact that there are several different hemoglobin genes is a bit confusing, and their placement apart from one another on different chromosomes is just an accident that forces medical students to do a bit more memorizing. But the evolution of a single hemoglobin gene into several different ones was vital to the development of mammalian species. Without them, we would still be sluggish worms.

The Switching of Human Hemoglobin

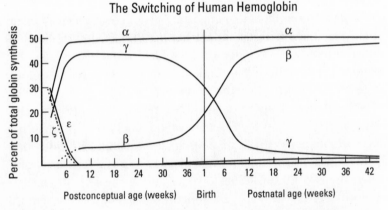

Figure 6 Shortly after conception, cells in the yolk sac of the fetus make red blood cells through expression of the globin genes zeta (ζ) and epsilon (ϵ). After about eight weeks of gestation, embryonic hemoglobin ($\zeta_2\epsilon_2$) is replaced by fetal hemoglobin ($\alpha_2\gamma_2$), which the alpha (α) and gamma (γ) genes together produce. Near birth the gamma genes gradually stop producing gamma chains, and the beta (β) genes dramatically increase their production of beta chains as partners for the alpha chains. The result is adult hemoglobin ($\alpha_2\beta_2$).

By capturing our med-student imaginations with examples of fascinating diseases like thalassemia and sickle cell anemia, our more skillful teachers were able to show us that the two chains of the hemoglobin molecule collaborate by gliding across one another during oxygen and carbon dioxide exchange. This remarkable interaction, they reminded us, demands a particular and unique amino acid sequence in each of the chains. The globin genes bear the responsibility for that sequence. Though mutations that change the sequence do occur, most are harmless. In fact, we know of nearly 500 abnormal human hemoglobins, the majority of which are clinically silent (that is, they cause no functional change in hemoglobin and no symptoms in the individual). They therefore are neither advantageous nor disadvantageous; they are merely polymorphisms that have arisen from time to time in communities around the world and have persisted in the local "gene pool" only when rates of intermarriage are high. They are usually discovered quite by accident when individuals are screened for abnormal hemoglobins.

Mutations of the alpha chain, while quite common, are usually without consequence. On the other hand, beta chain mutations, which are even more frequent than alpha mutations, more often produce a functional disturbance such as sickle cell anemia or the kind of thalassemia that afflicts Dayem. Those mutations would ordinarily disappear, since they do not favor survival and childbearing, were it not for the killing influence of malaria on those with normal hemoglobin genes. As "normal" infants are more readily killed by malaria, those with sickle trait or thalassemia trait are more likely to survive, thereby ensuring the concentration of the defective gene in the population.

After Ingram discovered that normal adult hemoglobin has two alpha chains and two beta chains, he carefully examined the same chains in sickle cell hemoglobin. He found what he was looking for in the beta chain. In sickle hemoglobin the amino acid called glutamic acid that normally resides in the number 6 position in the beta chain is replaced by another amino acid called valine. Since there are over 140 amino acids in the beta and the alpha chains of hemoglobin, it is difficult to understand how this single exchange could wreak so much havoc in the molecule. But the fact remains that this single substitution of one amino acid for another in a very long molecule causes the hemoglobin to elongate into a rod-like shape when it gives up oxygen. The rods of hemoglobin change the shape of the red cell into a sickle-like form. The sickle cells become rigid, block the circulation, and cause the many painful and debilitating manifestations of sickle cell disease. Twenty-five more years would pass before the specific DNA mutation that causes the substitution of valine for glutamic acid in the beta chain would be identified.

As soon as Ingram had defined the amino acid substitution in sickle cell anemia, he and others tried to demonstrate similar abnormalities that might help us to understand patients like Dayem with thalassemia. There, progress was very slow. Thalassemia is rarely associated with an abnormal hemoglobin, at least in the Mediterranean or Middle Eastern world. The total circulating hemoglobin may be very low (as it certainly was in Dayem), and there may be a relative if not absolute increase in fetal hemoglobin, but the residual adult hemoglobin (if there is any) is completely normal except in very rare circumstances. This fact strongly suggested that thalassemia must most often be due to a failure in the *regulation* of the total output of the beta gene, and not to a defect that alters the amino acid sequence of the protein. At the time of Dayem's visit, no one knew enough about the regulation of gene output to go further.

All we physicians could conclude in the fall of 1968 was that in severe thalassemics like Dayem, both beta genes are somehow defective. This is an innocuous mutation in fetal life, because in the fetus, gamma chains are attached to alpha chains to produce fetal hemoglobin. The fetus does not require beta chains. After birth, however, the gamma genes switch off and beta genes are supposed to switch on to produce beta chains, the adult partners for alpha chains. If both beta genes fail to turn on, the result is severe thalassemia (see figure 6 on page 32).

The disease is not obvious at birth, but it is readily apparent—as it became in Dayem—by the end of the first year of life. The severity of the disease, we were certain, must be directly proportional to the extent of the failure of the two beta genes to express themselves. Moreover, the severity of the disease must be moderated by the extent to which the activity of the gamma genes might persist. Beyond those simple conclusions, those of us working with thalassemic patients in 1968 knew next to nothing about the causes and possible cures of this disease, because we had no idea how beta and gamma genes work. We wondered, however, whether we could come close to a cure of the disease if we could prevent gamma genes from switching off after birth.

By the time Dayem arrived to see me, I had become fascinated by the thalassemia problem. The question was, could I apply whatever knowledge I had to help him and others like him, and could I make an impact on a disease that was better known in his part of the world than in my own?

JUST BEFORE DISCHARGE, Dayem's family and I had another long conference to plan his future care. It was the second of many meetings that I would have with Mrs. Saif during the next three decades to discuss Dayem's future, as well as a hundred other topics. It began my abiding responsibility for Dayem and my deep friendship with him and his family.

In that meeting I had to re-emphasize that we were now embarked on a very dangerous course. We had obtained a sample of Dayem's bone marrow cells and had stained them for iron. They contained only a bit more iron than the cells of an average six-year-old. But the course of transfusions that we were about to launch would inevitably choke his cells with iron, and the iron would kill him if we did not find a way to deal with it. Second, I could not be sure that his immune system would not become sensitized to red cell transfusions and begin to reject them. And finally, the blood preparations themselves might be contaminated with hepatitis virus or some other deadly agent. All of these were serious risks, and none could be excluded. But we all agreed that he could not go on as he had been.

Dayem rapidly improved during his first hospitalization, but the next dilemma was obvious. The Saifs would be living in Mexico, because of Mr. Saif's business responsibilities. How could we possibly supervise this boy's care in Mexico? We needed a pediatrician who could take over primary responsibility. Fortunately, Children's Hospital has regularly trained many foreign residents and fellows, and Miguel Herrera, an excellent pediatrician, was immediately called into service. When the phone line finally permitted, I explained the situation to him. Miguel—Mickey to us—never appears overwhelmed. He had not had much experience of thalassemia, but Dayem needed a good doctor, not an expert. We could supply the expertise. Mickey would provide the general pediatric skill and wisdom. Over a crackling and intermittently dead phone line, we forged the partnership that would be responsible for Dayem while his parents were in Mexico.

Mickey would see to it that Dayem was regularly transfused with red cells and that his general pediatric care was first class. He would report on the results of each transfusion and would try to phone us if there were any untoward complications. Dayem was not to engage in any strenuous activity until his bones began to heal and strengthen. We didn't want to deal with any more fractures in a boy whose heart function would soon improve enough to make exercise seem attractive to him. All of these conditions and all of the data were summarized in the first of many letters about Dayem that were sent to physicians wherever he lived—in Mexico, London, and Washington, D.C. During his peripatetic young life we always found a physician to take care of him while we supervised and organized the care from our small office at Children's.

Today, there is an international network of physicians who understand thalassemia care. Itinerant patients need to be encompassed by the network so that their care can be readily supervised and a rational long-term approach maintained. We hand off patients to one another like aircraft flight controllers passing individual planes from one FAA tower to another. We rely on one another for intelligent, on-the-spot decisions because a physician cannot practice sensible medicine without being face-to-face with the patient. The network becomes the eyes and ears that help pediatricians make individual decisions while the patient's coordinating physician establishes the overall policy. This approach works for the patient and establishes strong bonds among the physicians as well.

The Saifs quickly grasped the details of my transfusion plan and accepted its hazards. They were pleased with the arrangements for Dayem's care in Mexico, but in truth they never could entirely assuage the guilt and its attendant anxiety that intruded into their thoughts whenever they laid eyes on their son. Yet both of them were bolstered to a considerable extent by religious faith. Mr. Saif repeatedly referred to the will of God. Faith in a higher power clearly gave him extra strength as he dealt with the fateful decisions we were making. Mrs. Saif had faith as well, but it was more a faith in action and willpower. She seemed less apt to meekly accept what God would offer without a pitched battle.

That attitude was closer to my own. There was something about this young patient and his family that filled me with an absolute determination to win the battle against thalassemia despite the odds. And not just to win it for Dayem but for all the children in our clinic who were facing the same Catch-22.

I knew that if we could not come up with a way to rid Dayem's body of excess iron, the transfusion program would probably kill the boy before he was twenty. Any sensible person would have to accept the likelihood that the treatment program on which we now embarked would give Dayem about ten years of well-being that would then be followed by a slow, agonizing death from progressive heart failure due to iron overload. I understood all of that very well. But like Mrs. Saif, I just didn't accept it. "We'll have to find a way," I told her. "I don't know what it will be, but we'll have to find it. We will fight our way out of the corner."

I know it sounded like bravado, and perhaps this was unconsciously meant to help me as well as her. But I actually believed it. I was not going to lose this boy—not on my watch. We would have to find a way for Dayem and for the children like him. And if there was no way, we would have to invent one. Their cases were not going to remain solely in God's hands. We were going to take plenty of responsibility ourselves.

Seduced by Thalassemia

DURING THE BEGINNINGS of what would become a world-wide search for abnormal hemoglobins, I was living the dutiful life of a first-year Harvard medical student. For endless hours we would do innumerable experiments on the chemical reactions in the body that make hemoglobin suck up oxygen in the lungs and deliver it to tissues. There was little conversation about how the protein was made, because in the early 1950s so little was understood about the mechanisms of gene function. But while I was staring with glazed eyes at an obsolete machine that measured oxygen and carbon dioxide in blood, the revolution in genetics was beginning.

I came to Harvard Medical School with a strong interest in the delivery of health care to the urban poor of Boston and Cambridge because I had been a very active social worker during my Harvard College years. I saw the inequities of health care delivery with my own eyes, and I was determined to deal with them. Furthermore, I had a fairly weak background in the basic sciences. I had taken the survey courses in chemistry, physics, and biology required for entrance to medical school, but I had never done research nor thought about the subjects in depth. The excitement of discovery was unknown to me, but the lure of inquiry was in the atmosphere of Harvard Medical School.

During my second year of medical school, I ran across an interesting clinical problem. The neurologists and internists on the

Harvard Service at Boston City Hospital had described patients with liver disease who lapsed into coma when they ate meat and had elevated levels of blood ammonia. Could the ammonia be responsible for the coma? The idea of such intoxication from normal food fascinated me, and I launched into a research project on blood ammonia that occupied all of my free time. To my immense satisfaction, my results were actually published in a leading medical journal, and the methods I developed were used by two of the Harvard teaching hospitals to measure ammonia in the blood of their patients. The research bug had bitten me very hard. I began to wonder about my future plans.

When I graduated from medical school in 1955, I never seriously considered any future career idea other than the adult medicine group practice and clinic in East Cambridge that I had planned for years. My father objected. "Bend the twig," he would say. "Old trees just snap if you push them." But I moved with the crowd and became an intern at the Peter Bent Brigham Hospital, a Dickensian institution for adults that was closely affiliated with, and across the street from, Harvard Medical School.

These were the initial years of the federal government's influence on the training of physicians in the affiliated hospitals of leading medical schools. In the East, major teaching hospitals such as those associated with Harvard, Yale, Columbia, Cornell, University of Pennsylvania, Johns Hopkins, and Duke began to receive what would become a vast flow of dollars from the National Institutes of Health to carry out biomedical research, train young physicians to become academic specialists, and influence them to enter a career now called clinical investigation.

Our intern group was heavily swayed by the excitement of young faculty members who were beginning their careers in research. We hoped to emulate their remarkable knowledge of differential diagnosis and treatment and become full-time salaried clinical investigators like them. The private practice of either primary care or specialty medicine was not for us.

Clinical investigators are physician-scientists well trained in a clinical subspecialty such as cardiology, endocrinology, hematology, and nephrology (the study of kidney disease). But most important, they have further training in one of two other areas. The majority gain experience in a basic science, such as biochemistry, physiology, or molecular biology, that underpins their clinical field, and then they use the tools of this science to advance their knowledge of the fundamental basis of diagnosis and treatment. Others are further trained in epidemiology and biostatistics and make advances by analyzing the outcomes of new diagnostic or therapeutic procedures.

Clinical investigators therefore represent a relatively small but vital group of physician-scientists who devote their professional lives to research efforts that advance our knowledge of medicine. The group of patients they recruit to participate in their investigations are people being treated in the major teaching hospitals associated with United States medical schools. Their understanding of the scientific methods and biological principles that underlie clinical practice permits them to apply new basic scientific discoveries to the treatment of disease.

In the old Brigham and hospitals like it, the hospital facilities and the laboratories set aside for research by clinical investigators were primitive by today's standards. The hospital had been built prior to World War I in the old pavilion style—thirty beds to a ward, one intern on at night with one student nurse. A senior resident and a nursing night-supervisor were available somewhere in the hospital for consultation or hands-on help, but much of the clinical laboratory work done on patients at night was still performed by interns. Hospital budgets were very low. As an intern, my salary was $25 a month, and a young staff nurse earned less than $2,500 a year. The residents who supervised me received about $1,500 a year. Full-time faculty salaries were much lower than the incomes of practicing physicians. To be a clinical investigator and raise a family required an independent source of funds. Life was very difficult for those who did not have one.

During the late spring of 1956 when I was completing my internship, I received a phone call from Dr. Gordon Zubrod, then the Clinical Director of the National Cancer Institute (NCI), one of the National Institutes of Health (NIH) in Bethesda, Maryland. Zubrod wanted to know whether I would care to join the United

States Public Health Service and become a Clinical Associate at NCI for a two-year period. In the first year I would care for patients with cancer, and in the second year I could choose a laboratory and do clinical or basic research.

The alternative was to join the Army or Navy Medical Corps and go to Korea, where we were gazing hostilely at the North Koreans and the Chinese across the 38th parallel after our first shooting encounter with communism on the Pacific rim. Married and now the father of two small children, I took about twenty seconds to accept the offer. In the summer of 1956 I traveled with my family to Bethesda, a move that would irrevocably change my career.

IT IS SOMETIMES difficult to comprehend how much influence a handful of individuals can have on the course of an entire institution of government and on intellectual development. But in the case of the revolution that has occurred in biomedical science, one can ascribe the present world pre-eminence of American medical research largely to the efforts of four people. They were Dr. James Shannon, a physician with special training in kidney function and malaria treatment, who first became the Director of the National Heart Institute and, from 1955 to 1968, the Director of the National Institutes of Health; Congressman John Fogerty of Rhode Island and Senator Lister Hill of Alabama, both of whom strongly supported funding for NIH as a top priority in Congress; and the late Mrs. Albert (Mary) Lasker, a philanthropist from New York who organized public and medical testimony and put enormous pressure on Congress, particularly for the benefit of the National Cancer Institute but for all of NIH as well.

Prior to their efforts, NIH was a little-known research arm of the United States Public Health Service, with laboratories and various disease-related institutes located on a sprawling acreage in Bethesda that had been donated to the government by the Wilson family. Shannon, who was well trained in physiology and pharmacology, had profound insight into the potential role of basic science in the development of entirely new approaches to the treatment of severe, chronic diseases. With the help of the three others, he forged a mighty institution that quickly became the envy of the world.

It is instructive to recall for a moment how the discovery of antibiotics, vitamins, and hormones profoundly impacted the ideas of research-oriented physicians like Shannon. My grandfather and many of his generation disparaged doctors because they knew that doctors practiced largely by guesswork. Though diagnosis based on history and the accumulation of bits of physical evidence gathered from prodding and poking could be amazingly accurate, treatment other than surgery was limited and arbitrary. Doctors didn't charge much in those days, and they came to the house (practices for which many people are still somewhat naively nostalgic), but the chance that a patient would actually benefit from the encounter was rather low.

Antibiotics, vitamins, and hormones changed all that. Here were simple molecules which, properly applied, could make vast changes in a patient's well-being. The death rate following streptococcal sepsis and pneumococcal pneumonia was markedly reduced by penicillin. The ghostly pallor and neurologic damage of pernicious anemia were completely reversed by one or two injections of vitamin B_{12}. A form of devastating diarrhea that decimated troops in the tropics could be totally alleviated by a few doses of the vitamin folic acid. Insulin saved the lives of diabetics.

These new approaches to diagnosis and treatment convinced Shannon and a few others that much more knowledge was about to come. They concluded that a massive attack on cancer, heart diseases, genetic disorders, and other intractable illnesses should be mounted. The attack would require an expansion of research both within NIH and in the nation's medical schools and their affiliated hospitals. Armed with the political skills of Fogerty and Hill and the ceaseless prodding of Congress by Mary Lasker, Shannon made it happen. Between 1955 and 1968 the NIH budget rose nearly 24 fold, from 81 million to 1.9 billion dollars, and today has reached the extraordinary level of over 10 billion dollars. It has continued to rise even in the face of domestic budget cut-backs that have plagued United States agencies during the past twelve years. Only in the past several years has it begun to plateau in constant dollars.

Perhaps the most important event in the Shannon years was the creation of Building 10, the Clinical Center on the NIH campus. Shannon designed this 337-bed research hospital to have beds on one side of the hallway and laboratories on the other, so that a continuous interaction of the laboratory with the patient could occur. The Clinical Center represented a massive federally supported expansion of an idea that had its beginnings thirty to forty years earlier at Rockefeller University and had been emulated on a smaller scale in such places as the Boston City Hospital's former Thorndike Unit and Massachusetts General Hospital's Ward 4, both affiliated with Harvard Medical School. In medical units like these, patients with diseases of interest to clinical investigators could be admitted and remain for days, weeks, or even months at no charge if they would agree to participate in studies designed to understand the physiologic or biochemical basis of their disease.

For example, in a particularly famous study, Dr. William Castle admitted patients with pernicious anemia to the Thorndike Unit for experimental treatment that lasted for weeks. Every day the number of new red blood cells (reticulocytes) that emerged from the marrow into the peripheral blood was estimated. Reticulocyte production failed to increase on a diet of raw meat (which contains Vitamin B_{12}) alone, but sharply increased when gastric juice—which Dr. Castle obtained from his own stomach—was added to the meat meal. This proved beyond question that intestinal absorption of Vitamin B_{12} from meat requires a substance in gastric juice that Castle called intrinsic factor. Patients with pernicious anemia do not produce intrinsic factor because the stomach cells that normally make it die off. Much later it was shown that this atrophy is due to an attack on the cells by an abnormal population of immune cells. Therefore pernicious anemia is one of the autoimmune diseases—diseases caused not by the immune system's failure to suppress an infection from the outside but by its overzealous attack on the very body it's supposed to be defending. This was the kind of new and exciting information that could be gathered only in such clinical research units.

It appeared to Shannon that a large federal effort to carry out clinical investigation on the NIH campus would greatly stimulate the flow of new medical information and train many physicians in the required techniques. To accomplish his goal, Shannon needed to revolutionize the NIH structure. First, he had to build a research hospital where there had been none before. Second, he had to staff that hospital with enough young doctors to care for patients night and day. Third, he needed to provide a major expansion of research resources for the leading academic medical centers, university-affiliated teaching hospitals, and basic science institutes so that graduates of the NIH training programs would have a place to work after they completed their tours on the NIH campus. He also needed to make an NIH career attractive enough to retain many of the very best and brightest of the young people within the NIH laboratories and in the Clinical Center. Amazingly, Shannon did it all. He is surely the father of the burst of activity in clinical investigation that flourished in the United States from 1955 to the present.

Today, careers in clinical investigation are no longer as attractive to young physicians as they were when I entered the field—for several reasons. First, young doctors no longer need to go into the Public Health Service to avoid the military draft. Second, more young physicians in training are married with families, in part because salaries of interns and residents have increased one hundred fold. They do not wish to move around. If they choose a career in clinical investigation, they tend to remain in the academic environment in which they received their clinical training and are less likely to travel to Bethesda.

Third, finances play an increasingly major role in the decisions of these young physicians. They begin their careers in deep debt because college and medical school tuitions have increased so much during the past two decades. Years spent at low pay are not appealing to them. A young impecunious clinical investigator can readily abandon a full-time and relatively low-paying academic career and open a private office to practice his or her clinical specialty in one of the suburbs that surround the large cities in which the major academic medical centers are located. This has two negative effects on academic medicine, beyond depriving it of bright young investigators: it puts more expensive specialists out into the community and unnecessarily raises health care costs, and it cuts off the flow of patients to the academic medical center, thereby reducing both its efficiency and its research capacity.

In the 1950s when I went to NIH, there were only a few academic medical centers in the United States that could possibly absorb the flow of biomedical research dollars and trained investigators that emanated from Washington and Bethesda. These centers had a finite growth capacity. Had policymakers been willing to enlarge these established centers and create only a few new ones, the research budget would have kept up with demand. But Americans are afflicted with a chronic need to grow, and in the last two decades medical facilities have expanded even more than football teams. Many so-called medical centers, replete with residency training and research programs, sprang up all over the country in one congressional district after another. Every congressman wanted a teaching hospital, with its flow of federal grants, in his district. There has been no, or very little, regional planning because Americans abhor regulation.

Today we see the inevitable pain of such unbridled growth. The NIH budget has begun to decline, and funds for the support of research and for the maintenance and renewal of research laboratories are very difficult to obtain. The infrastructure of our best laboratories needs repair, but money is not available, and bright young people are having enormous difficulty funding their projects. We are downsizing, but we are creating grave uncertainty and poor morale in the process.

In the meantime, fierce competition for research grants has arisen from a flood of Ph.D.-holding graduates of basic science training programs who are strong competitors for NIH grants, and whose scientific experience is not "diluted" by clinical training. Why not let the basic scientists do the research, it is argued, while the physicians care for the patients? The answer is quite simple. The goal is to improve the quality of medicine. One needs a broad array of talents to solve the problems posed by disease. We need basic scientists *and* clinical investigators to collaborate with one another. The problems posed by stubborn illnesses like inherited diseases, cancer, and AIDS require the efforts of both. But the competition for funding remains grim and creates a great deal of uncertainty about the stability of a future career based on research productivity.

Clinical investigation as a profession has also changed somewhat because of the advent in the 1980s of molecular medicine, an approach to diagnosis that does not require a patient in a bed but only a sample of his or her cells. If the next step in molecular medicine—so-called gene transfer therapy—becomes a practical reality, there will be a resurgence of research on patients in the hospital as physicians try to find ways to insert a gene into the particular affected organ. The development of clinical centers for molecular medicine, particularly human gene therapy, will certainly require the collaboration of basic and clinical investigators.

All of these concerns and uncertainties were in the future, back in July of 1956 when I stepped as a lieutenant into the United States Public Health Service. For the first time in my life, I was going to earn a respectable living, and receive excellent training as well.

M Y INITIAL assignment was to care for children with leukemia under the aegis of Emil Frei and Emil Freireich, two physicians with similar names and somewhat similar personalities who were recruited by Zubrod to improve the results of cancer therapy, particularly in children. They introduced combination chemotherapy on both the adult and the pediatric cancer units at NCI. Though they were often derided as "kooks" or even described as heartless by those who believed that their efforts would be useless at best, and toxic and agonizing at worst, they and a few others who were similarly minded persisted. When I started to work with them as a Clinical Associate, there were no survivors of childhood leukemia. Today, between 60 and 70 percent of children with that disease are cured. Granted, some suffer serious side effects of chemotherapy and radiotherapy, but they survive, and that progress began on the wards of the Clinical Center at NIH.

After nearly a year of patient care duties in the Cancer Institute, I was instructed to join the laboratory of Dr. Nathaniel Berlin, who had recently been recruited by Zubrod to NCI. Berlin is an experimental hematologist interested in the production of red cells. I had no interest in hematology or red cells. I wanted to study ammonia toxicity in liver disease.

Berlin, a small man who could fold himself in a Buddha-like fashion into a government-issue office chair, rocked back and forth and listened to me beg for release from red cells to work on ammonia. Finally, he responded, "Tell me, if we were in uniform, how many stripes would I have on my sleeve?" I knew he was the equivalent of a Navy captain, so the answer was four. "And how many would you have?" he asked. "Two" was the correct response. "That's why you're going to be a hematologist and work hard on red cells this year," he explained. "If you also want to work on ammonia, you can do it evenings and weekends, but weekdays you are working *here* for the U.S. Public Health Service in *this* lab with *me*. You are going to become an expert on red cells, so start to enjoy it."

I often think of that scene when residents and fellows come to me for advice about their careers. They have many options and often don't know which one to take. They are never ordered around. How easy it is to be ordered into a field. There are no doubts at all! Of course, I went home in a rage, but within a few weeks I found myself getting deeper and deeper into what became my "chosen" field. I shared the laboratory with two of my Harvard Medical School classmates, Thomas Waldmann and Sherman Weissman. Both of them went on to illustrious careers in immunology and molecular biology, respectively, Waldmann at NIH and Weissman at Yale. Weissman later made very important contributions to the solution of the thalassemia problem at the molecular level.

Next door was a metabolism laboratory to which another clinical associate, Daniel Nathans, was assigned. Later he shared the Nobel Prize for discovery and initial application of the enzymes in bacteria—called restriction enzymes—that break DNA into pieces. None of the molecular medicine that is done today, and none of our knowledge of the molecular basis of thalassemia, would be available without that discovery. Weissman, Waldmann, and Nathans are but three among hundreds of examples of what Shannon's program accomplished for U.S. and world medicine.

The year in Berlin's laboratory at NCI sped by. During those months, I learned many of the tools of red cell research that I would use in subsequent years. In July of 1958 I returned to the Brigham house staff for one year to complete my training requirements for certification in internal medicine.

One day in the spring of 1959 a patient was admitted to my service at the Brigham who was to change the direction of my career. Mr. Zhangi was a 70-year-old retired fruit peddler from the North End, a district of Boston in which many Italian immigrants live. He complained that he was becoming deeply yellow, and he had mild but definite pain in the upper right side of his belly. Inspection revealed that Mr. Zhangi was indeed extremely yellow, and underneath the yellow color he seemed very pale. Below the left rib cage there was a long well-healed scar that seemed to be quite old.

"What's the scar, Mr. Zhangi?" I asked.

"I don't know, doc. Dr. Jones had me operated on a long time ago. I have been fine ever since."

"Where's Dr. Jones?"

"Oh, he's probably still over at Mass General. I haven't seen him since the operation. That was in 1920."

I pressed for details but got no useful responses. The scar looked like the kind that would have followed removal of the spleen. Could that be related to Mr. Zhangi's pallor and yellow color? There was something else that was peculiar about him. He was short, his forehead seemed prominent, and his nose was broad. In some ways he resembled an elderly, albeit spry, chipmunk.

But it was his blood counts and the appearance of his red blood cells that startled me. Mr. Zhangi was certainly anemic. His blood hemoglobin concentration was half of normal. Under the microscope, his red blood cells were grossly abnormal. At least half of them were nucleated like the red cells of birds. Most of them were very pale and contained little hemoglobin. They looked like flat plates, and they contained flecks of debris that I knew represented bits of nuclei and granules of iron.

Now when an elderly man shows up in a hospital looking deeply yellow and anemic and complaining of pain in his abdomen, there is one overwhelmingly likely diagnosis—bleeding cancer somewhere in the gastrointestinal tract with obstruction of the bile flow from the gall bladder. It's a sign of a terminal case. But Mr. Zhangi was spry. He was bothered by his color and the mild abdominal pain, but he hadn't lost weight, and, above all, his blood tests showed that he was not iron deficient from chronic bleeding. Indeed, there were granules of extra iron in his red cells.

A better diagnosis, though an incredible one, was that Mr. Zhangi had thalassemia, and that, after a lifetime of excessive red cell destruction and compensatory red cell production, in which he produced a large amount of bile pigment from the rapidly destroyed red cells, some of the pigment had precipitated in his gall bladder and formed stones. One or more of the stones had finally lodged in and partially blocked the large duct that collects all the bile pigment from the liver and dumps it into the gut. In short, Mr. Zhangi had gall stones of an unusual variety—pigment gall stones—and they were doing what gall stones often do: obstruct the duct and cause jaundice.

When I reported my findings and diagnostic ideas to the chief resident and suggested that we call in the surgeons to explore Mr. Zhangi's duct, he looked at me with a mixture of irritation and pity.

"Look," he pointed out, "you don't make a diagnosis of thalassemia for the first time in a 70-year-old man. That disease is diagnosed in childhood. The patients have to be transfused for all of their lives. Are you crazy? This guy has been peddling fruit all over Boston. He had one hospitalization nearly forty years ago. He's been in great shape ever since. How can you say that he's got thalassemia?"

"Because his red cells say so under the microscope, and look at this plasma." I had centrifuged Mr. Zhangi's blood. The plasma wasn't just yellow. It had the tell-tale greenish brown color that accompanies very rapid red cell destruction. Even the urine was brown. Some of the excessive pigment in the plasma was leaking through Mr. Zhangi's kidneys into his urine.

But my trump cards were the x-rays. They were astonishing. Mr. Zhangi's skull film was very abnormal. The two plates of skull bone that contain bone marrow were widely separated by what must be an excess of bone marrow volume. The marrow spaces of the upper arms and upper thigh bones were massively expanded.

The outer edges of the bones were so thinned by the expanded marrow space that it was surprising Mr. Zhangi had never had a fracture. The chest x-ray was the most startling. The rib marrow space was strikingly expanded, the heart was big, and on both sides of the vertebrae there were huge masses of tissue that looked like metastatic cancer.

The chief resident looked first at the films, and then witheringly at me. "Look, Nathan. Look at the films. The guy is riddled with cancer. He's got it all over his bones and it's spread to his lungs. Forget about thalassemia. Look at those red cells again. You've made a mistake. He's got cancer. It's bleeding and it's spread all over him!"

My chief resident was then, and is now, a terrific doctor. He practices in Birmingham, Alabama, and he's one of the best doctors in the South. But I knew cancer from my two years at the National Cancer Institute, and this wasn't cancer. I had spent the past year learning about red cells. This man had all of the findings of thalassemia, including the chest x-ray. I was convinced that the masses along the vertebrae represented lumps of bone marrow that had been squeezed out of the confined space in the vertebrae like toothpaste and had found room to grow in the gutters alongside the vertebrae in the chest. The bones that to my chief resident looked riddled with cancer were actually separated by expanding bone marrow.

To prove it, I took a sample of Mr. Zhangi's blood over to Children's Hospital next door. There worked one of the foremost pediatric hematologists in the world, Louis K. Diamond. While Dr. Diamond opened and read his mail, I presented the case of Mr. Zhangi and showed him the x-rays and the blood smear. Dr. Diamond finally laid down the envelope opener. "This is certainly thalassemia," he said, with impressive authority. "We'll measure the fetal hemoglobin. It will be very elevated."

"Hemoglobin researchers are getting very excited about some new ideas that your chief resident hasn't heard about yet. Mr. Zhangi has what some of my colleagues are starting to call thalassemia intermedia. Both of his beta globin genes are functioning poorly, but for some reason he's making a lot of fetal hemoglobin, so the total production of hemoglobin in his red cells is much better than it is in the usual garden variety of severe thalassemia. That's why it's gone unnoticed all these years. Does he have children? If he does, they will all have thalassemia trait."

I said that Mr. Zhangi had never married. "Well, you can't have everything," said Dr. Diamond. "But he can still teach you a lot. You see, beta thalassemia comes in many forms. The most common type is one in which both beta genes are totally or almost entirely functionless. They make either a very small amount of beta globin or none at all. If a child inherits two of these genes, one from each parent, that child is going to have severe thalassemia and require transfusions for the rest of his life. Less commonly, a thalassemia gene may be quite moderate or even very mild. Some beta globin chain is produced by that gene. Thalassemia intermedia can occur when the child inherits two thalassemia genes but at least one of them is moderate or mild, or when a lot of fetal hemoglobin is made. Those patients can be surprisingly free of severe signs and symptoms, particularly if both beta thalassemia genes are of a mild type."

"Tell your chief resident that he's wrong. And by the way, I'll ask Miss Neveska in the hematology lab to do the fetal hemoglobin right away. I'm interested myself." He returned to his mail while I sat there. After a few minutes of silence, I realized that the interview was over. I walked back to the Peter Bent Brigham lost in thought.

The next day Dr. Diamond called me. "We were right," he chuckled. "Mr. Zhangi has about 80 percent fetal hemoglobin. The rest is normal adult hemoglobin. You better come over and chat some more."

I ran across the bridge between the Brigham and the Children's that day, little realizing that I would cross it permanently seven years later.

Dr. Diamond had obviously read his mail already. He was poised to teach. "What you've got to understand about Mr. Zhangi is that your chief resident isn't *entirely* wrong. Mr. Zhangi doesn't have the common severe beta thalassemia that is seen wherever malaria was present in the old world. Those children die if they don't get transfused because the defect in their beta genes is so severe. They make almost no adult hemoglobin. In fact, the only hemoglobin they do make is fetal hemoglobin, but they can't make enough of it to survive."

"So why does Mr. Zhangi have so much hemoglobin F?" I asked. "Normal adults have a tiny amount of fetal hemoglobin in the blood. For example, Miss Neveska says I have only 0.5 percent hemoglobin F. Now that's 0.5 percent of 14 grams of hemoglobin per hundred milliliters of blood, or only 0.07 grams of fetal hemoglobin per hundred milliliters. Mr. Zhangi makes 80 percent F and has 7 grams per hundred milliliters of total hemoglobin. That's 5.6 grams of hemoglobin F per hundred milliliters, or 80 times more F than I have. How does he do it?"

At that point, Dr. Diamond himself looked puzzled. "I can't tell you why right now," he said. "And don't forget, he makes quite a bit of normal adult hemoglobin, too. Twenty percent of 7 grams per hundred milliliters is 1.4 grams of hemoglobin A per hundred milliliters. That's nowhere near what you and I make, but at least one of his beta genes is not totally knocked out. It can make some normal beta globin. The other one may be knocked out completely, but somehow his gamma genes are functioning at a very increased rate. That's another reason why he has thalassemia intermedia. He can make much more total hemoglobin than can the child with severe disease. We're going to have to learn much more about how the hemoglobin genes influence one another to understand this more thoroughly. But before you leave, tell me something. You said that a Dr. Jones over at Mass General told Mr. Zhangi to have the operation on his abdomen in 1920. Could that have been Chester Jones?"

I laughed. As usual, Dr. Diamond was way ahead of me. I had requested the MGH record. The record room promised to get it quickly, but hospital records, particularly old ones, move like tortoises.

Meanwhile, the surgeons came to see Mr. Zhangi. They had never heard of thalassemia in an adult, particularly in a 70-year-old adult, but they and my chief resident now agreed that Dr. Diamond was very likely to be correct—even if I was suspect. They operated on Mr. Zhangi and removed a bunch of pigment stones from his duct. They also took out his gall bladder. His yellow color rapidly disappeared.

Six days later, the Massachusetts General Hospital record arrived. There were the legible notes of the intern who admitted Mr. Zhangi to the MGH medical service in 1920. The intern's name was Chester Jones. That name may not be remembered very much today except around the MGH and Harvard Medical School, but Chester Jones became one of the best gastroenterologists in the country. He and his colleagues Walter Bauer, Paul Dudley White, and James Howard Means had made the MGH medical service world-famous. Jones was one of the great clinical teachers of the Harvard Medical School. At that time, he was still very active.

The notes in the record made it clear that Jones, the intern, had missed Mr. Zhangi's diagnosis. That was understandable because thalassemia was not described in the clinical literature until five years later, in 1925, by Drs. Thomas B. Cooley and Pearl Lee. They reasoned that the five patients they described must have some form of congenital anemia (an anemia apparent at birth), but they did not think it was inherited because the parents were not severely anemic. Following Cooley and Lee's report, there were many similar descriptions, and it became generally known that the disease was present largely in individuals whose races originated on the shores of the Mediterranean. Today thalassemia is also known as Mediterranean anemia or Cooley's anemia.

In 1932 Dr. George Whipple, who was Dean of the University of Rochester School of Medicine, carefully described the pathology of thalassemia and gave the disease its name. Dr. David Weatherall, one of the world's leading investigators of thalassemia and the author with Dr. John Clegg of a classic textbook on the subject, describes how this occurred as he learned it from Dr. George W. Corner, who was at Rochester with Whipple when he was doing his early pathologic studies of Cooley's anemia.

Dr. Corner tells the story like this. "Because I was perhaps the most bookish of the young Rochester faculty, Dean Whipple made me his informal consultant on literary matters, several times asking my opinion on questions of nomenclature and etymology. Wishing to avoid the eponymic title *Cooley's anemia,* Whipple sought a name that would associate the disease with the Mediterranean area, all the cases known at that time having occurred in families originating there. He had studied Greek at Phillips Academy, Andover, and he recalled the great story in the Anabasis of Xenophon's army coming over the mountain, and gazing at last at the sea, the ten thousand shouting as one man, 'Thalassa, thalassa!' Whipple sent for me, and asked whether I thought the name *Thalassic anemia* correct and appropriate. I had, in fact, never studied Greek, but of course I knew of the retreat of the Greek army from Persia and could at least tell the Dean that both words of his proposed name were from Greek roots, and therefore properly associated. I gave no thought to the geographic aspects of the problem. Not until long afterwards did I learn that the view, hailed so joyfully by the homebound Greeks, was actually the Black Sea. The weary men still had a voyage before them, and the Bosphorus to pass before reaching the Mediterranean Sea."

Weatherall, in recording his conversation with Corner, went on. "As it turns out, however, the minor classical uncertainties of the Rochester School do not matter. Recent work suggests that the Black Sea is a very suitable location to give its name to thalassemia; it is (unlike the Mediterranean) surrounded with the disease on all sides!"

"By the late 1930s the clinical syndrome of thalassemia had been well described. However, the idea that it was a genetically determined disorder was not formally proposed until the paper of the Greek clinician, Caminopetros, was published in 1938. Interestingly, however, descriptions of the heterozygous state for thalassemia [thalassemia trait] had appeared in the Italian literature as early as 1925, though it was fifteen years before it was realized that the condition which was described by the early Italian writers was related to the disorder seen at the same time in the United States by Cooley."

Obviously, the young intern Jones would have no way of knowing of all these developments in 1920. He ascribed Mr. Zhangi's condition to what was then known as Banti's syndrome. Guido Banti was an Italian pathologist who lived from 1852 to 1925. He described enlargement of the spleen secondary to alcoholic liver disease. That form of splenomegaly was regularly associated with anemia in part because the large spleen trapped the red cells. Alcoholic liver disease, perhaps due to excessive wine drinking, was much commoner than thalassemia in Banti's day, and today, in the United States, remains a much more common cause of splenomegaly than is thalassemia. So Jones, that great diagnostician, missed the diagnosis. The splenectomy was carried out for purported Banti's syndrome. Mr. Zhangi disappeared into the streets of Boston to peddle his fruit and was never seen again by a physician until he appeared at the Brigham forty years later.

Dr. Jones later came over to the Brigham to visit with Mr. Zhangi, who recognized him at once. Displaying amazing recall, Dr. Jones described all the details of his decisions on Mr. Zhangi, as the two of them enjoyed a reminiscence of an incorrect diagnosis made nearly forty years earlier that preceded a successful treatment.

A FTER Dr. Jones left and Mr. Zhangi was discharged, I continued to ponder the disease. I was particularly bothered by the variation in the amounts of fetal and adult hemoglobin that could be found in the blood of different patients. Mr. Zhangi had a lot of fetal hemoglobin in his blood, whereas most patients with the severe form had much less. The difference seemed arbitrary. I began to read as much as I could about the disease and consulted extensively with the many experts in the Harvard and MIT community.

Perhaps, I thought, I might improve my understanding of thalassemia by examining families. As luck would have it, Dr. Diamond told me of a fascinating patient he had seen—a child just like Mr. Zhangi but with 100 percent fetal hemoglobin.

"Here is an interesting family, Dr. Nathan. Both the mother and the father have thalassemia trait. They have one normal beta gene (β^A) and one beta thalassemia gene (β^T). They each have 10 grams of hemoglobin per 100 milliliters of blood. But there's something very interesting about the mother. She has 12 percent fetal hemoglobin with a total hemoglobin of 10 grams per 100 milliliters, and the father has only 1 percent fetal hemoglobin with the same total hemoglobin. Now, let's look at the offspring. This family had only one child. He has seven grams of hemoglobin per 100 milliliters of blood and very abnormal red cells. He clearly has thalassemia, but it's relatively mild, and he has 100 percent fetal hemoglobin. He's like your patient Mr. Zhangi, but he has even more fetal hemoglobin" (figure 7).

"There's only one reasonable explanation for this. Clearly the child inherited both thalassemia genes from his parents, and both thalassemia genes must be associated with a complete loss of normal beta chain production because the child has absolutely no adult hemoglobin. However, the thalassemia gene that he inherited from his mother, who has 12 percent fetal hemoglobin, must be associated with high and persistent gamma chain production while it also prevents any normal beta chain production. The father's beta thalassemia gene makes no normal beta chains either, but it is not associated with increased hemoglobin F production. So while this child cannot make any adult hemoglobin, he is saved by the fact that he has an enhanced gamma chain factory—the persistent gamma gene or genes that he inherited from his mother. The combination of the stress of the anemia, the fact that the gene associated with beta thalassemia in the mother induces gamma chain production to make fetal hemoglobin, and, finally, the fact that the beta genes of the mother and the father are totally non-functioning has produced this tremendous effect on fetal hemoglobin accumulation."

"I can't tell you why some patients with beta thalassemia express a great deal of fetal hemoglobin and others do not. It's going to take a lot of work to understand this, but we have to classify this mother as an individual with what I would have to call high F-beta thalassemia gene. She makes a very large amount of hemoglobin F in her own cells. When she passes on her high F-beta thalassemia gene to her offspring, who is anemic because he also inherited a severe beta thalassemia gene from his father, even more F is made. The child has mild to moderate thalassemia because of all that hemoglobin F production. We have to understand the basis of the control of hemoglobin F synthesis. If we could get other patients with the ordinary kinds of thalassemia to make more F, they could be helped a great deal."

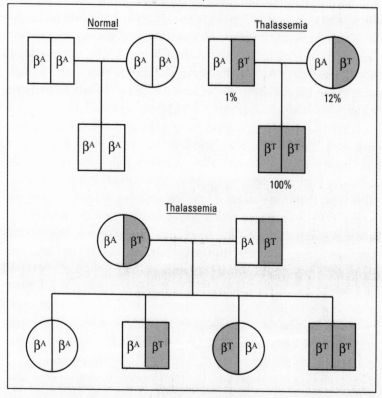

Figure 7 In a family (top left) where the father and mother each have two normal beta genes ($\beta^A\beta^A$), all of their children will be normal. In a family (bottom) where both parents have thalassemia trait (one β^T gene), with each pregnancy there is a 25 percent chance of producing a normal child ($\beta^A\beta^A$); a 50 percent chance of producing a child with thalassemia trait ($\beta^A\beta^T$, $\beta^T\beta^A$), and a 25 percent chance of producing a child with severe thalassemia ($\beta^T\beta^T$). In the family described to me by Dr. Diamond (top right), the father and the mother each had thalassemia trait, and the mother had a markedly elevated level of fetal hemoglobin (12 percent). The child had the misfortune to inherit both thalassemia genes, but he also inherited his mother's capacity to produce fetal hemoglobin; therefore his red cells contained 100 percent fetal hemoglobin.

I sat there fascinated. One of Mr. Zhangi's parents must have had a beta thalassemia gene that was associated with no hemoglobin A production but with high hemoglobin F production. Unlike the family described to me by Dr. Diamond, the other Zhangi parent must have had a beta thalassemia gene that made a small amount of hemoglobin A, because Mr. Zhangi had 80 percent hemoglobin F and 20 percent hemoglobin A.

From that meeting, I came away with something very important. Beta thalassemia genes must be of three types. A common type makes no beta chain at all. Another type, perhaps equally common, makes a small amount of normal adult beta chain. A third type makes no normal beta chains, but a large amount of hemoglobin F is produced by its accompanying gamma genes. Today, we call the first type "beta zero" thalassemia, the second type "beta plus," and the third type "thalassemia intermedia." As is often the case in life, much depends on who your parents are.

I slowly walked back across the bridge to the Brigham, my head swimming with thoughts about the many thalassemia syndromes. I was still somewhat confused, but thoroughly seduced. I would plunge into the thalassemia problem as soon as I could.

Grasping
Opportunities

INEVER SAW Mr. Zhangi again. He vanished into the North End of Boston just as he had disappeared following the removal of his spleen at the Massachusetts General Hospital in 1920. But my interest in his unusual form of thalassemia remained strong. When my senior residency was completed in 1959, Dr. Frank Gardner, then chief of hematology at the Brigham, offered me a tiny laboratory where I could devote much of my attention to anemias, and particularly to inherited disorders of the blood.

Though the space was terribly cramped and the equipment of variable sophistication, I began to make some progress. Through Gardner's efforts, I was fortunate to receive a fellowship from the Medical Foundation, a local research organization initiated by the United Way of Massachusetts. Suddenly my income rose from $1,500 to $7,500 per year. Even my parents thought I had a real job at long last. Gardner was himself awarded a research grant from the National Institutes of Health. That paid for a technician to help me in the lab and for necessary supplies.

I'm not sure that I would describe our group as classical researchers. We might more aptly be described as medical science opportunists. We were not necessarily trying to answer basic biological questions, but were responding to the issues raised by the patients we saw in the clinic and on the wards.

One day, Park Gerald, a member of Dr. Diamond's staff and the discoverer of several important abnormal hemoglobins, called to tell me that he knew two adults with beta thalassemia of moderate to intermediate severity. They needed some medical attention and were too old to be cared for at Children's. Was I interested? "Interested" was a vast understatement. I leaped at the chance. Soon Stephen D. and John C. became my patients. I gave them free medical care in return for their willingness to give me blood samples for my research.

Stephen D. was a sheet-metal worker who lived about twenty miles from the hospital. As a child, he had undergone a splenectomy for an anemia that was poorly characterized. Years after the operation, a sample of his blood was obtained by Gerald, who made the correct diagnosis of thalassemia intermedia. Gerald found him to be anemic with many circulating nucleated red cells and typical thalassemia-like red cells. His blood contained at least 40 percent fetal hemoglobin. The rest was hemoglobin A.

John C. was a plumber who lived in East Boston. He had been mildly anemic all his life, but he was drafted into the army and was medically discharged only when his large spleen was detected. John's hemoglobin was not very low, about 10 grams per 100 milliliters, but at least 30 percent was fetal hemoglobin. He too had thalassemia intermedia.

The influence of all that fetal hemoglobin on the behavior of red cells in the circulation piqued my curiosity. Could fetal hemoglobin be protective of red cells in some way then unknown? Was the life span in the blood of red cells rich in fetal hemoglobin longer than the life span of those containing very little? To answer these questions, I joined forces with Tom Gabuzda, one of my medical school classmates who had just arrived as a new member of the hematology group at the Brigham. Tom is now chief of hematology at the Lankenau Hospital outside of Philadelphia. Together, we formulated a research plan to study these two cases of thalassemia intermedia.

Our plan, as I explained to Stephen and John, was to give them a tiny dose of an amino acid (glycine) which had been tagged with a radioactive tracer (called an isotope). The glycine would travel to the bone marrow, where it would be taken up by their newly formed red cells and incorporated into both adult and fetal hemoglobin. We would measure the radioactivity that appeared in the blood when the red cells carrying those labeled hemoglobins emerged from their birthplace in the marrow, and we would follow that radioactivity for three or four months until it disappeared. This would tell us whether the two hemoglobins had different or identical survival rates. A longer survival of the fetal hemoglobin would suggest that fetal hemoglobin was "packaged" in its own special red cells and that those cells were somehow protected from destruction.

The experiment was safe, I told them, but it would not in any way improve or cure their condition. It would also be inconvenient: somehow we would have to meet to draw a blood sample twice a week for four months. Since Stephen couldn't afford to miss a day of work, I proposed to meet him early in the morning in the parking lot of a large shopping mall near his worksite. With this arrangement, he wouldn't have to go out of his way. Stephen readily agreed to participate. So did John, who lived closer to the hospital and agreed to come to the lab to have his blood sampled.

The experiment began. In our collaboration, it was Tom's task to set up a system that would separate hemoglobin A from hemoglobin F in each blood sample. My major job was to design a method of measuring the tiny trace of radioactivity in the many hemoglobin samples that Tom prepared. Neither task was routine in those days. The radioactivity measurement was particularly difficult. For safety, the dose of labeled amino acid given to John and Stephen was necessarily very low. The peak amount of radioactivity that accumulated in their blood was only slightly above that of the natural background radiation (microwaves which emanate from all parts of the universe and can be detected in almost any environment on earth). Each sample had to be individually burned to reduce it to carbon dioxide and water. All of the radioactivity was in the carbon dioxide. The gas had to be trapped and counted in what was then the first "liquid scintillation" radioactivity counter in the hospital.

The counter, a sensitive detector of very-low-level radioactivity, was the second model of its kind to be manufactured in the United States. Since we had not yet entered the transistor era, the machine contained over a hundred radio vacuum tubes, most of which had to be monitored carefully to minimize background radiation "noise." I learned a lot about vacuum tubes, and spent much of my spare time in radio repair shops searching for the correct ones. As more counters were delivered to the hospital and the medical school, I became an amateur repairman, wandering from laboratory to laboratory with my trusty tube tester. Fixing broken liquid scintillation counters became an art form.

My other unusual task was to slip into a shopping mall parking lot in the early morning, sit next to Stephen in his car, and obtain a blood sample without being observed or spilling any of it on the seat cushions. On one occasion, I failed to notice that a state police car had driven into the mall right behind me. Just as the needle entered Stephen's vein, the state cop pounded on the car window, gesticulating wildly. The motions were obvious—get out of the car, and don't make any sudden moves. Fortunately, I had decent identification and avoided a nasty fracas in the state police barracks. Stephen was unfazed. We continued to meet at the mall, but we kept an eye out for curious onlookers.

The results of the experiments were remarkable. Hemoglobin F survived in the circulation far longer than hemoglobin A. This provided incontrovertible evidence that hemoglobin F protects the red cells in people with beta thalassemia. Tom Gabuzda and I reported our initial findings in a letter to the journal *Nature,* and more completely in two subsequent articles in the *Journal of Clinical Investigation.*

With such an encouraging start, I decided to try to understand the phenomenon in greater detail because of its therapeutic implications. If patients with beta thalassemia could be influenced to make more hemoglobin F, their anemia and the high turnover of their red cells could be improved. But before I could dream of manipulating fetal hemoglobin production in patients, I would have to have much more information about *how* fetal hemoglobin actually protects the thalassemic red cell.

Those initial studies took place in the early 1960s. Now, thirty years later, it is useful to reflect on the ethics of this kind of patient investigation. Both John and Stephen were in their thirties, married, and the father of small children. They were intelligent men, but neither had a college education. They knew very little about medicine, but they knew I was deeply interested in their disorder and in their well-being. When I asked them to participate in the experiments, I knew it would be inconvenient for them, but I was certain that it would do them no harm; the Atomic Energy Commission had licensed me to administer this radioisotope in this particular form at this dose to normal humans. I was also certain that the data to be gained would be informative.

Since I had no evidence of any risk and, above all, since I saw myself as their medical advocate, I did not notice a conflict of interest in the relationship that had the potential to undermine the quality of their decision. It was true that medical science would benefit from the experiment. Indeed, the three papers that emerged from the studies that Tom Gabuzda and I performed have been repeatedly cited and are considered important contributions to our understanding of thalassemia even today. It's also true that I did not act alone. The experiment was planned very openly, and all of my colleagues in the Division of Hematology, including the division chief, were well aware of our plans and approved them unconditionally. Stephen and John were carefully informed in detailed conversations with me, and they were reassured that I would respond to them whenever they needed me.

But there was a flaw in the procedure of informed consent because I was not a disinterested party. True, no harm was done, and the medical literature benefited, but so did I. The results of a lot of hard work were three important papers in prestigious journals and several presentations at professional meetings that brought me, a relative unknown, wide recognition in the field. I received praise and requests for reprints from around the world. The head of the Department of Medicine at the Brigham began to notice me as an up-and-coming young clinical investigator. If that continued, it would lead to election to select societies, promotion, and a higher salary. To claim that someone in my position was acting solely as his patients' advocate would be naive if not disingenuous.

It pains me to write this now. It is painful because I truly did not see the conflict of interest at that time. I was utterly convinced that I had only Stephen and John's welfare at heart because I was completely committed to them as patients. They knew that I would never do anything knowingly to hurt them, and to this day they are very loyal to me. However, Stephen and John did not benefit directly from those experiments, and I did. I should not have been solely responsible for gaining their consent, and the method Tom and I used to assure that our patients understood the risks, whatever they might be, was inadequate.

Not too many years later, egregious examples of unethical and even dangerous clinical investigation began to be recognized. One of the first to speak out on the issue was Dr. Henry Beecher, the chief of anesthesia at Massachusetts General Hospital. The events that led the United States Public Health Service to conduct a long experiment in which penicillin was deliberately withheld from African-Americans infected with syphilis shocked the medical establishment and the nation. Congress stirred, and the NIH established independent review boards within each grantee institution to oversee all clinical investigation.

Today, if I wished to conduct my experiment on patients like John and Stephen, I would have to apply for permission from my institutional review board. The required documentation of safety and efficacy would be extensive. The patients would have to read and sign an informed consent document that would have first been examined in detail by the institutional review board and probed carefully for any misleading statements, particularly understatement of risk or (in the case of therapeutic research) overstatement of benefit. Absent the complete permission of the independent institutional review board, I would not be able to conduct the experiment on hospital property—and if I flouted the system, I would be denied future NIH grants and would probably lose my faculty position.

Institutional review boards not only protect patients from overzealous physicians, but also protect physicians from their own errors of judgment. It's very easy for a physician to fall into the trap of self-approval. Following the discovery of antibiotics, physicians have been widely accepted as bearers of the contributions of medical science to the public. Even my grandfather and his generation of suspicious doubters, who saw physicians as lazy mendicants drinking their coffee and doing nothing useful, would welcome the modern scientific physician. But it must be said that the social status physician-researchers enjoy outside the hospital, and the deference of patients and staff within it, can sometimes lead to an arrogant lack of caution.

Only recently have doctors begun to slide into unpopularity again. In large part this is because many doctors, in their zeal to deliver high-technology care, have failed to maintain an old-fashioned personal warmth in their relations with patients and their families. Physicians are also seen as being very well off while medical care costs skyrocket, plunging the nation further into debt while many citizens go without adequate health care. Ask the car dealers in any small city to whom they sell the most expensive cars, and too often they'll say it's to the bankers, the lawyers, and the doctors. Today, for example, even full-time academic physicians are far better off financially than they were when I was investigating Stephen and John. They don't do nearly as well as procedure-driven specialists in private practice, but they are comfortable if they are not overly burdened by tuition debt. In the "bad old days" we were still pretty threadbare. So threadbare, in fact, that one of my patients, an elderly Jewish tailor, took pity on me. One day, after I completed my examination of him in the cramped office that served our entire group, he got off the exam table and asked me to stand by it while he measured me for a pair of pants. When he returned with them two weeks later, it was like a scene from a Woody Allen film. I put on the pants and swam in them.

"Vell—ve'll tek 'em in a liddle."

Poor Mr. Bornstein—he was a terrible tailor but a lovely, generous man. He knew I wasn't going to buy any clothes on my salary—so he did what he could to correct the situation.

In some respects, those were better days for the doctor-patient relationship, and certainly for physician/investigator–patient/subject relationships. The patient/subject saw the physician/investigator as an advocate who had no financial stake in the outcome, and as a member of an economic class not vastly different from his own. "Hi doc" was the regular greeting. It was a greeting between equals—people of equal income, if not education. Today, we have separated ourselves from most of our patient/subjects not only intellectually, by dint of our professional and technologic training, but also as a result of our relative salary advantage. I'm not suggesting that academic physicians should return to the impoverished days of the late 1950s, but if top academic compensation begins to approach that of private lawyers, we may be seen by members of the U.S. Congress (most of whom are lawyers living on comparatively modest government salaries) as being only slightly less acquisitive. If that perception takes hold, we may lose the public support that we must have if biomedical research is to flourish. The NIH budget must not be viewed as a jobs program for wealthy doctors. The compensation for research physicians should be reasonable but on the modest side if public support is to be its mainstay.

W HILE I WAS CONDUCTING my investigation of the survival of fetal and adult hemoglobin in the blood of Stephen and John, I regularly saw them for any medical problems they might encounter, and I repeatedly studied their blood through electrophoresis and microscopic examination. Both patients remained moderately anemic—John with about 30 percent fetal hemoglobin and Stephen with about 40 percent. The remainder was hemoglobin A. In that respect, they were very much like Mr. Zhangi. At least one of their two beta genes must have been functioning, albeit at a reduced rate, and one or more of their gamma genes that produce the gamma globin chains of fetal hemoglobin must have been very active.

Under the microscope, Stephen's blood cells looked very much like those of Mr. Zhangi. Most had the appearance of broad, flat dishes with a thin rim of hemoglobin coating the edges. The minority were somewhat smaller, more normally shaped, and contained much more hemoglobin. These cells, we learned a bit later, were rich in fetal hemoglobin. Stephen's cells were also striking in another way. They contained a great deal of foreign rubbish. There were many that retained intact or fragmented nuclei; a high proportion were burdened with large granules of iron; and there were barely visible chunks of some material that I couldn't identify. The flat, pale cells that lacked fetal hemoglobin were particularly laden with rubbish.

John's cells were very different from Stephen's. Though they also varied in the amount of fetal hemoglobin they contained, they did not seem to be burdened with debris, and many of the cells seemed to come to a point; they looked like large teardrops.

I kept wondering why the cells of these two men looked so different if they had the same diagnosis and roughly the same hemoglobin level. Then a simple clinical fact occurred to me. Stephen, like Mr. Zhangi, had had his spleen removed, whereas John's spleen, though enlarged, remained in the upper left section of his belly. Therefore, John and Stephen might give me an opportunity to evaluate the effects of spleen removal on the red cells of patients with thalassemia. Could those lumps of vaguely staining debris in Stephen's cells be related to the removal of his spleen?

As I wondered how to make those lumps more visible, I recalled that similar aggregates appear in the red cells of patients with another inherited anemia found in malarious parts of the world. When these patients take certain drugs such as antimalarials, compounds like chlorox form in their red cells; then lumps appear and their red cells are rapidly destroyed. In that disease (which is due to an inherited deficiency of a red cell enzyme called G6PD), the lumps contain damaged hemoglobin, and there are special stains that outline them very clearly. I ran across the bridge to Children's Hospital to see Josephine Neveska, the experienced technician in the hematology laboratory who had helped me with Mr. Zhangi's blood analysis a year or two before. I was sure that she would have a stain that would help me see these lumps in Stephen's cells more clearly.

"John and Stephen," she responded. "I know their blood very well. Dr. Diamond asked me to look at it many times. I'll be happy to do special staining for you."

Josephine Neveska was one of those marvelous technicians trained when the microscope was the dominant diagnostic tool in hematology and the ability to perform perfect staining of cells was the most important skill in the clinical laboratory. Rapidly and expertly, she stained the smears of red cells with special dyes and returned them to me to take the first look. I was amazed at what I saw. John's cells were smooth and free of any lumps at all. Stephen's were laden with large lumps of violet-staining rubbish that seemed to sit on the inside of the red cell membrane and distort it. In a moment I realized that Stephen's cells were full of hemoglobin lumps—damaged hemoglobin that had precipitated within the cells.

Normal hemoglobin is tremendously soluble; red cells can hold more than 30 grams of hemoglobin per 100 milliliters of red cell water. That is the equivalent of one ounce of protein in three ounces of water. It has the consistency of glue. Normal hemoglobin will not precipitate within red cells to form lumps unless it is badly damaged, as in the anemia that people with G6PD deficiency develop after taking antimalarial drugs. Could that explain the difference? Was Stephen G6PD deficient and John not? I asked Ms. Neveska to screen them both for the protective enzyme. The results were as I suspected. Both had entirely normal levels. The precipitated hemoglobin could *not* be due to enzyme deficiency.

Then I had a bit of insight. Perhaps *both* of these men had hemoglobin precipitates in their red cells, but John's intact spleen was constantly removing them. The spleen is, after all, the carpet sweeper of the blood. Red cells that enter it are literally grasped by rubbish-cleaning cells and licked like ice cream cones until their rough external edges are smooth. If there are any free lumps inside, they put their tongues in and suck them out, like a child finding a chocolate chip in a scoop of ice cream. When the splenic cell has finished its cleansing job, it usually spits out the red cell, now in better shape from the encounter. However, if a red cell contains very large pieces of rubbish, the splenic cell may have to hold it in its mouth a bit longer than usual and suck in quite a bit of cell to remove the lump. That may leave the cell looking quite elongated. Red cells that carry junk and have such a brush with splenic cells can look like teardrops when they are finally cleaned out and return to the circulation (see figure 1 on p. 13).

If my ideas were correct, all spleenless patients with thalassemia would have red cells that looked like Stephen's, while patients with intact spleens would have red cells that looked like John's. With Josephine's help, I could solve that issue rapidly. Children's Hospital has a large thalassemia clinic because Boston has a fairly substantial Italian population in its North End and in East Boston. I asked Josephine if she would do special staining on the red cells of a few spleenless patients and of a few whose spleens had not been removed. Within a week she had the information. My hunch was correct. The lumps of precipitated hemoglobin were seen only in the spleenless patients. Those with intact spleens had teardrop-shaped red cells like John's. The next question to investigate was obvious: Why would hemoglobin precipitate in the red cells of patients with beta thalassemia?

Sometimes one is very lucky in research, and the right idea hits you when you least expect it. One of my great clinical teachers, Samuel A. Levine, a famous cardiologist of his day, gave me some advice that I've never forgotten. "When you have a patient with a difficult diagnostic problem," he said, "worry about him all the time. Think about him while you're at dinner; think about him in the shower; don't let him out of your mind. The right idea will come to you if you keep the problem in your mind." I was staring at Stephen's red cells, as I had done for days, when I suddenly noticed something interesting. The lumps were much larger in the large flat red cells that had very little hemoglobin in them than in the well-filled fetal-hemoglobin-containing cells, some of which had no inclusions at all. Suddenly the whole problem seemed ridiculously simple. The lumps must be made up of unpaired alpha chains!

If that was true, then beta thalassemia is not simply a failure to make the beta chains of hemoglobin. It is also a toxic disease—a disease that develops when some part of the body is being "poisoned." In the case of thalassemia, the poison is the unmatched alpha chains. The chemical nature of these free alpha chains is such that they immediately fall out of solution in the cell if they don't find suitable beta or gamma chain partners with which to form hemoglobin molecules. As the free alpha chains rapidly precipitate, they damage the red cell membrane and leave the cell to the not-too-tender mercies of the rubbish-eating cells in the marrow and in the spleen. If enough free alpha chain is made, the poor red cells are gobbled up by rubbish eaters as soon as they are produced in the marrow. On the other hand, if the cell makes a great deal of gamma chain, the alpha chains find the gamma chains as dancing partners, combine with them to form fetal hemoglobin, and do not precipitate. That's why the cells containing fetal hemoglobin look so healthy, and that's why patients who can make more gamma chains have mild or moderate disease: first, they have some decent hemoglobin to carry oxygen around; and, second, the gamma chains soak up the alpha chains that would otherwise poison the cell and force it to die in the marrow or elsewhere in the circulation such as the spleen or even the liver, where rubbish-eating cells also abound.

I was hot on the trail of a new concept, and I was getting very excited. Thalassemia is not merely a deficiency disease; it is a disorder of unbalanced protein synthesis. Hemoglobin is comprised of two pairs of different chains that must form a four-chain molecule. If one partner is not formed, the unmatched member will poison the cell. Beta thalassemia is very severe because free alpha chains are so terribly unstable and destructive.

Next I needed to look at some examples of alpha thalassemia. At the time there were relatively few patients with alpha thalassemia in Boston because the disease is more common in Asians than in Italians, and the wave of immigration from Southeast Asia to the northeastern United States had not yet begun. There are four nearly identical alpha globin genes in normal individuals—two on each chromosome 16. Mutations of those genes involving complete deletion of one or two of them on one or both chromosomes are seen in Italians and Greeks but are more common in Chinese, Vietnamese, Cambodians, Laotians, and Indonesians. Complete deletion of all four alpha genes is fatal. Fetuses with this deadly lesion are almost always stillborn. Deletion of three of the four alpha genes causes a surprisingly mild form of thalassemia. The individual red cells contain low amounts of hemoglobin, and they are destroyed somewhat rapidly in the spleen and elsewhere, but the resulting anemia is not very severe, and transfusion is rarely required. There are excess beta chains in the red cells, as expected, but they don't cause as many problems as excess alpha chains do. Having an insufficient number of alpha chains with which to dance, four of these free beta chains will cling together to form an abnormal and poorly functioning hemoglobin called hemoglobin H. We call that type of thalassemia "hemoglobin H disease." I wondered whether the beta chains that accumulate and form hemoglobin H gradually precipitate in the cells and cause the accelerated red cell destruction that characterizes the disease.

I called Park Gerald to ask him whether he knew of any patients with hemoglobin H disease. Being the local expert on thalassemia, he had screened the blood of many patients, and he immediately told me about Tony R. and another family of patients with hemoglobin H disease. Fortunately for me, one of them had had his spleen removed. I couldn't wait to look at the blood. Sure enough! The spleenless patient had the expected precipitates in some but not all of his cells. Later I realized that the unmatched beta chains are much more soluble than are unmatched alpha chains. When they form four-chain molecules with one another, they temporarily stay in solution. Eventually, however, they precipitate, damage the cell membrane, and cause the accelerated destruction of the cell.

Of course there were several more refined experiments to do to clean up the theory and make the case for unbalanced hemoglobin synthesis airtight, but the important observations and the insight came from looking down the microscope at those cells and thinking about the problem in the context of particular patients. With the help of Robert Gunn, a bright young Harvard medical student, who later became head of the Department of Physiology at Emory University, I published my concept of thalassemia as a consequence of unbalanced hemoglobin synthesis.

There was one small problem. Careful review of the literature showed that I was not alone in my thoughts. A Greek hematologist named Phaedon Fessas, who was to become chief of the First Medical Service at the University of Athens, had made very similar observations. In fact, he was the first to prove by chemical analysis that the inclusions observed by both of us contained hemoglobin, and he was the first to propose that in beta thalassemia the inclusions represent precipitates of alpha chains. So I wasn't the only one to come up with the idea. But I was one of two, and that had to be good enough. Later, Phaedon and I became fast friends. He and his colleagues have made many very important contributions to the field on a tiny research budget, proving that research of high quality depends primarily on brains and secondarily on money (though of course some money is rather important).

While Bob Gunn and I were putting the finishing touches on our paper on unbalanced hemoglobin synthesis in thalassemia, another thought occurred to me. The body must have several ways to improve the balance of production of globin chains and reduce the impact of free alpha chains. First, the defect in beta chain production might be mild, and therefore not many alpha chains would have to go without partners. Second, increased gamma chain production might provide partners for the excess alpha chains, in which case fetal hemoglobin would be the result. Finally, some people might inherit not just defective or missing beta genes but defective or missing alpha genes as well. Because one or more defective alpha genes would reduce the production of alpha chains, these patients might actually have milder disease as a result. Even though they could not make much hemoglobin in their cells, what they did produce would be more balanced. Thalassemia intermedia might be caused by any one of those three options.

To evaluate these potential causes, I would need to have better methods of measuring the production of the alpha, beta, and gamma globin chains in red cells. Fortunately, David Weatherall and his colleague John Clegg, both of whom are now at Oxford, had developed a very useful method for separating all of the globin chains and measuring the rate at which they are made in the developing red cell. They did this while they were research fellows at Johns Hopkins. It isn't a particularly easy method, but the technique works; and in the right hands, it is very reliable.

Using Clegg and Weatherall's approaches, I began to explore the concept of imbalance in thalassemia in a careful fashion. I discovered that the three methods of amelioration that Bob Gunn and I had proposed could actually be detected in patients. It was particularly exciting to demonstrate that alpha thalassemia could partially correct the damage done by beta thalassemia. Working with Yuet Wai Kan, who joined the laboratory a year or two later, I gathered substantial evidence that John had a milder disease in part because he had alpha *and* beta thalassemia defects, while Stephen was protected because he could make large amounts of gamma chains and had a relatively mild defect in beta chain production.

B Y   T H I S   T I M E, I was becoming nearly obsessed by the thalassemia problem and by inherited blood diseases in general. Just then, Dr. Diamond announced that he wished to retire and move to California, where his children resided. I was asked whether I would like to move to Children's Hospital from the Peter Bent Brigham, become a pediatrician, and devote myself to pediatric hematology. For a little while, I wrestled with the idea because I couldn't see how I would master pediatrics, particularly general pediatrics, after a decade of training in internal medicine. An interview with the head of the Department of Pediatrics at Children's dispelled most of my fears. Charles A. Janeway was one of the great leaders of American pediatrics. An expert in immunology and infectious diseases, he too had been an internist at the Brigham and had crossed the bridge to Children's because he had become fascinated by the inherited susceptibilities to infection that are observed almost exclusively in children. He assured me that I could learn enough pediatrics to be a useful member of the staff, and that there were some marvelous pediatricians at Children's who would be happy to coach me if I was willing to learn.

I made my final decision because of many long conversations with another mentor, William B. Castle, the physician who had used his own gastric juice to discover intrinsic factor (the protein responsible for the absorption of vitamin B_{12}). Where Dr. Castle sits, it was said, is the head of the table. Dr. Castle asked me whether the idea of becoming a pediatrician made me happy. I answered that it certainly did, but that most of my friends thought it was terribly risky. Suppose, they said, that I find I'm not skilled enough to diagnose and treat small babies and children? I would then be relegated to a minor role in an advancing clinical field.

In his laconic voice, Dr. Castle gave me this advice: "I know a lot of people who are not satisfied, but keep doing the same thing because they aren't willing to take chances. If the idea of pediatric hematology makes you happy, you should do it."

"I agree with Bill Castle," announced Dr. Diamond, when I reported that conversation. "You know, years ago when Dr. Kenneth Blackfan was chief of pediatrics here, he encouraged me to give up the general practice of pediatrics to join his department as a pediatric hematologist. It seemed very risky at the time. There were no pediatric hematologists anywhere, and the idea of being an employee of Harvard and the hospital didn't look very good financially. But I wanted to do research and teach, and there was no other way to go. So here I am—I survived. You will too."

That same day I had a second long interview with Charles Janeway. The meeting allayed nearly all of my concerns about the value of such a change, but created another one. Dr. Janeway had certainly made the transition, but he was extraordinarily intelligent. Did I have the intellectual capacity to make the move and continue my own productivity? By the end of the discussion there was no turning back; I knew that I might fail, but I had to take the chance. With the example of Janeway in front of me, and the supportive prodding of Diamond and Castle behind, I crossed the bridge to Children's for the last time.

The transfer of my small laboratory from Peter Bent Brigham to Children's in 1966 took about a day to accomplish. A couple of us trundled the equipment over and set up shop in a confined space in the basement of a structure that would soon support a new ambulatory clinic building. The hospital laundry was next door. My office was a 5 × 6 foot cubicle in a corner of the lab. The lab's only microscope was kept there as well. For some reason, a modern edition of a Victorian water closet was fastened to the wall above my head. Water intermittently flushed down a clear plastic pipe attached to it. I never did ask where that water came from, what it contained, where it was going, or what its predictive significance might be. I didn't really want to know. This was the first private office I had ever had. True, only one other person could fit in it, and it had no door, but it was *my office*. I could sit there alone with my thoughts, interrupted only by the flushing water closet.

Fortunately, tucked into other corners of the laboratory were some wonderful young physicians who came to study thalassemia with me. Among my first colleagues was Eli Schwartz, who is now professor of pediatrics at the University of Pennsylvania and pediatrician-in-chief at the Children's Hospital of Philadelphia. Another was Kan, who years before had been a member of our group at the Brigham, where he had made it his business to marry my best lab technician, Alvera Limauro, before taking a job in Montreal. There, he became interested in thalassemia. He returned from Canada to Philadelphia and then in 1967 decided to join me at Children's.

By that time my former technician was the mother of a baby girl and refused, despite my entreaties, to return to the lab. I never quite forgave Kan for stealing her. Alvera insisted, quite rightly, that individuals have a right to marry whom they choose, have children when they choose, and work when and where they choose. I told her that I agreed in principle, so long as exercising those rights didn't interfere with laboratory work! Kan is now the Louis K. Diamond Professor of Laboratory Medicine at the University of California in San Francisco, an investigator of the Howard Hughes Medical Institute, a member of the National Academy of Sciences, and one of the leading medical geneticists in the country. In 1991 he won the Lasker Award, the most prestigious prize for research in the United States—frequently a prelude or postlude to the Nobel Prize.

A year or so after Kan returned to Boston, we were joined by Bernard Forget. Bernie was a McGill graduate and had also been at NIH. Later, he became chief of hematology in the Department of Medicine at Yale. We were all quite cramped in our small laboratory, but this was the era of great expansion of academic biomedical research in the United States. NIH grants for construction of new laboratory facilities began to flow like a river into universities and research hospitals. Children's Hospital was the fortunate recipient of a large grant to construct a new research laboratory building to be named for John Enders, a Nobel Prize-winning scientist at Children's who was the discoverer of methods that led to the development of the polio vaccine.

By 1970 our group was comfortably ensconced in a whole floor of a wonderful new laboratory space named in honor of Dr. Diamond. We could take on new colleagues, approach new problems, train more young people, and make room for the equipment we would need to explore problems at a fundamental level. We plunged ever more deeply into thalassemia.

By the time of Dayem's first visit, I was completely immersed in the problem.

Hard Choices

WHEN DAYEM was discharged from Children's Hospital on September 23, 1968, at the age of six and a half, he carried with him a detailed letter of instructions to Mickey Herrera in Mexico to transfuse him again six weeks later. On the sixteenth of October, the first of many letters arrived from Mrs. Saif.

"First of all," she wrote, "I would like to tell you that your friend Dayem is at an English school and that he is more than happy. The principal of the school and the teachers seem to be very comprehensive [sic] and willing to collaborate. Dayem has even a meal at this school, and it does not seem to tire him at all. The smile and the laughter he brings back home every day are enough to convince anybody."

It was wonderful news. Despite the risks, this boy who had never before spent a single day at school was now having a decent life. The question before us was how to maintain it, and we began to consider bone marrow transplantation.

The concept of marrow transplantation for the treatment of human blood diseases has been with us for nearly four decades. The clinical field began in 1957 with the pioneering work of E. Donnall Thomas, now in Seattle. Two years later, a French hematologist treated some lethally irradiated survivors of a serious atomic reactor accident with marrow cells obtained from co-workers. The results were unsatisfactory. The marrow cells of the donors were rejected by the immune cells of the recipients.

As a procedure, marrow transplantation is relatively uncomplicated. A donor is anaesthetized and a large needle is inserted into his or her pelvic bone. A syringe is attached to the needle and marrow cells are sucked out. The procedure is repeated until about a pint of marrow cells and blood is collected. The cells are then given by vein to a compatible recipient who is suitably prepared to receive them. If all goes well, the donor marrow cells make their way to the recipient's marrow, where they start producing blood cells.

In most marrow transplants, the donor and recipient must be immunologically compatible with one another. Identical twins are fully compatible, and about one out of four siblings share a great deal of immunologic compatibility. When donors are not sufficiently compatible with recipients, the transplanted cells may be rejected or they may attack the tissues of the recipient and cause a terrible illness called graft-versus-host disease.

In 1968, marrow transplantation was a highly dangerous procedure for the recipient—one being carried out in only a few places in the world. Much of what we know about this therapy is owed to the work of Don Thomas. He came from Texas to Harvard Medical School and went on to the Peter Bent Brigham Hospital as an intern and resident, where he became fascinated by the early efforts in that hospital to develop a successful approach to kidney transplantation. His interest in hematology was stimulated by his chief resident, Clement Finch, who soon thereafter became the chief of hematology in the new medical school that had been formed at the University of Washington in Seattle.

In the initial kidney transplant attempts, before the so-called immunosuppressive drugs had been developed, rejection occurred in every case. The physicians involved realized that they would have to find a way to deal with graft rejection or they would never be successful with organ transplants. Many techniques were tried. In one series of experiments, the Brigham group, prior to transplanting a kidney, irradiated the entire body of the recipient and then transplanted bone marrow from the prospective kidney donor into the patient. It was hoped that these drastic preliminary steps would reduce the immunologic capacity of the recipient and make him capable of accepting a subsequent kidney graft from that same donor. The procedure didn't work. None of the approaches of that era could sufficiently reduce the barriers to organ grafting. Nevertheless, the attempt to transplant marrow excited Don Thomas. He believed that with sufficient work and a few breaks, he might be able to master marrow transplantation, while he left the kidney transplant problems to others.

Though Thomas was one of the finest clinical teachers I have ever known, his research received little encouragement at the Brigham. No one was interested in bone marrow transplantation, largely because there was no space in which to pursue the required work. If he was to explore that field, he would have to go elsewhere.

Elsewhere proved to be the Mary Imogene Bassett community hospital in Cooperstown, New York. In that unlikely venue, a puckish, irreverent iconoclast named Joseph Ferrebee was also interested in marrow transplantation. Thomas and Ferrebee began to work on the procedure using beagles as their experimental subjects. They would irradiate a dog, suck marrow cells from the bones of a litter mate, and then transfuse the marrow cells from the donor beagle to the irradiated one. If the transplant took, the irradiated beagle would survive; if not, the dog would die of radiation disease. The idea was to keep doing experiments until one worked.

This approach had been adopted by Paul Ehrlich when he undertook the search for an antibiotic that would kill the spirochete that causes syphilis. Ehrlich developed an animal model of syphilis and made one chemical compound after another, trying each of them in the animals until the 606th one worked. The drug was an antimony-containing compound that was later called Salvarsan, but was dubbed "606" when it was first used in practice.

Ehrlich's plodding step-by-step approach was distinctly out of favor by the time that Thomas joined Ferrebee. Most of his colleagues thought Thomas had lost his senses and would soon be forgotten in the wintry woods of upstate New York. For years he and Ferrebee labored on with the beagles and actually did some successful marrow transplants, but the successes were rare. Later they realized that simple Mendelian genetics controlled the rejection process. Experiments carried out in France, England, and the

United States showed that a cluster of genes organized on chromosome 6 actually define immunologic compatibility and control graft rejection. Each individual has two clusters, one inherited from each parent, and there is a 25 percent chance that two children of the same parents will have inherited the same sets of clusters and be relatively compatible with each other with respect to organ transplant. Each could donate a solid organ like a kidney or a liquid organ like marrow to the other with a much lower risk of rejection than if incompatible siblings or unrelated individuals were the donors.

Even when beagles with compatible marrow were used as donors, Thomas observed that there was a very high risk of failure of engraftment or rejection unless the ability of the recipient to reject foreign tissue was temporarily suppressed with drugs or unless the donor-recipient pair were identical twins. Since identical twins are very rare, a great effort had to be made to develop a safe and effective schedule of drug administration and total body irradiation that would prepare a recipient to accept a graft.

Surprisingly, Thomas and Ferrebee were able to make progress in this complex field, and they slowly worked their way up to human marrow transplantation. They restricted their initial clinical experiments largely if not completely to patients with leukemia or other immediately fatal diseases, because the transplant procedure was itself apt to be fatal and they did not wish to contribute to the death of the patients who had come to them desperate for a last chance at life. Despite the advances in beagles that Thomas had made in Cooperstown, his clinical accomplishments with human patients were very meager. When he moved in 1963 to join his old mentor, Clement Finch, in Seattle, he received very little encouragement from his peers.

At that point almost everybody thought that human marrow transplantation was not feasible. Not only was rejection a serious problem, but the very effort to control it created yet another difficulty. In order to prevent rejection, drugs and radiation have to be used to lower the capacity of the recipient to fight off the foreign cells, but the same cells that destroy the transplanted marrow cells are also responsible for killing germs. Patients treated with enough drugs or radiation to accept a marrow graft frequently succumbed to overwhelming infection.

Furthermore, there was a third menace awaiting recipients of transplanted organs. If the graft took, and if the infections were successfully treated, the immunity-producing cells of the donor soon began to circulate in the recipient and pose a very dangerous threat to the host. Though the transplanted donor cells may share many of the genes of the immunologic compatibility cluster with those of the recipient, they remain different in nonidentical individuals. Invariably the engrafted cells begin to see the host as foreign and to attack the recipient as if he is the foreign invader. The result is graft-versus-host disease, an immune disorder characterized by persistent eczema, diarrhea, liver failure, and lung disease. Don Thomas invested a lot of effort developing ways to prevent or treat this terrible outcome, but in 1968 when we were contemplating marrow transplantation for Dayem it was already one of the procedure's most dreaded complications. It remains so today.

In the late 1960s, my colleague Fred Rosen and I began to use marrow transplantation to treat infants with a very rare immunologic disease called severe combined immune deficiency (SCID). Fred was the chief of the Division of Immunology at Children's. In SCID, infants are born with an inherited failure to produce the marrow cells that are responsible for the immune response. They cannot produce any antibodies, nor can they produce the cells that directly attack invading organisms. And while they also cannot reject organ grafts, if they receive even a simple blood transfusion they will die of overwhelming graft-versus-host disease because the foreign immunity cells in the transfused blood grow in them and kill them. Obviously a marrow graft is very tricky in such children. If they are given too small a dose of marrow, it will not grow. If the dose is too large, they will die of graft-versus-host disease.

Rosen and I treated a few of these SCID patients, and then, encouraged by Thomas's work (for which he eventually received the Nobel Prize—in 1990), we went on to transplant patients with leukemia or aplastic anemia. We also decided to try to treat another rare inherited disorder called the Wiskott-Aldrich syndrome (WAS), a disease named for the individuals who described it. WAS is an unusual disease. These children have defective immune systems, but they still have immunity cells and can reject grafts. They also produce defective platelets that are abnormally small and do not plug up vessels well. Hence the patients are apt to bleed very seriously. Those with severe disease are afflicted with eczema (because their abnormal immunity cells attack their skin cells), and they bleed badly into the skin when they scratch their itchy rashes. Their lives are miserable and usually very short.

Like thalassemia or leukemia, WAS is a disease of the blood-producing cells in the marrow. All blood cells are derived from a tiny population of stem cells that grow and differentiate into the separate marrow cell lineages that include the red cells, white cells, platelets, and immunity cells. To cure WAS, leukemia, aplastic anemia, or thalassemia, one needs to wipe out all of the defective stem cells that give rise to the unwanted cells and replace those stem cells with normal compatible ones that do not carry the defect. If the defect is inherited, like WAS or thalassemia, the donor cannot be an identical twin because such a twin would have the same disease. The only suitable donor is a compatible sibling. There is a one-in-four chance that any sibling may be compatible. Very rarely, a parent is compatible. Fritz Bach and his colleagues in Wisconsin had accomplished a partially successful marrow transplant in a WAS patient in 1968.

Our treatment of WAS with bone marrow transplants turned out to be excellent. Eventually we were able to cure 90 percent of our patients, and they are healthy, growing children today. In the United States generally, over 85 percent are cured. The others die of complications such as drug reactions, graft rejection, overwhelming infection, and graft-versus-host disease. Some might properly ask how we could find such a record gratifying or even acceptable. After all, nearly 15 percent of the patients in the United States die from the complications of the procedure that is intended to cure them, rather than from their own disease. Our answer to that is that we have chosen the lesser of two evils. We are certain that nearly *all* of the patients who have been grafted would have died of their disease within two years had we not treated them. We are confident that, on balance, we and our colleagues in other centers have made the right decision.

OBVIOUSLY thalassemia was very much on our minds in the late 1960s as the immune deficiency experience was being gained. Our new patient, Dayem, might prove to be a perfect candidate for marrow transplantation. He required constant red cell transfusion and was therefore at serious risk of death from iron overload within a few years. Why not take the risk of transplantation? He had at that time at least a fifty-fifty chance of dying from the procedure itself a decade before his heart disease would be expected to kill him, but if he survived the transplant, he would gain a lifetime.

It was my responsibility to determine whether the procedure might be an option in Dayem's case. I asked Mickey Herrera to draw blood on all of the family members so that when Mrs. Saif and Dayem returned for an evaluation, they could bring the blood samples with them. With those samples we would test to see whether any family member might be a compatible bone marrow donor. The test results were disappointing; none of the family members was sufficiently compatible to serve as marrow donors, and we were forced to abandon the idea for Dayem.

Today, in certain rapidly fatal disorders, we have begun to use unrelated donors who match the recipients in the tests for compatibility, but the results are much worse than those that we achieve when sibling donors are used. Though I might have recommended a marrow transplant for Dayem had a sibling donor been available, I would not consider an unrelated donor for him. I would not have let my own frustration and worry about his future dominate my judgment. One cannot threaten patients with a therapy that one knows to be almost certainly fatal. If patients have insuperable difficulties, the physician can't eliminate the problem by planning a therapeutic execution. I knew that then, and I know it even more certainly now.

I often recall that attempt to cure Dayem with a transplant when I consider the many conversations I have had with parents and patients about risk-taking in therapy. There are some physicians who argue that if a patient has an ultimately fatal disease, a major risk of early death should be taken in an effort to achieve a permanent cure. I largely agree with that position, but one has to have a very clear idea about what one means by the term "ulti-mately fatal." I have no hesitation about advising marrow trans-plantation for certain fatal illnesses such as severe immune deficiency or acute leukemia because those diseases are normally lethal a year or so after diagnosis. Severe thalassemia is also ulti-mately a fatal disease, but when we initiated Dayem's chronic transfusion program, we could expect survival of at least ten years. Our dilemma was that we were quite certain he would become progressively ill after seven or eight years of transfusion. Therefore, we entertained the idea of marrow transplantation for him and considered accepting the hazard of his early death, because we believed that we would probably gain less than ten years of good life with conservative transfusion therapy. On the other hand, we realized that marrow transplantation carried a very high risk of failure and fatality, and in the end we concluded that the task before us was to establish a new treatment program that would extend his productive life without taking such an immediate mor-tal risk. We were confident that the art and science of marrow transplantation would improve with time. If we could keep Dayem with us, a new and safer transplant approach might be developed.

Since we considered transplantation for Dayem, there have been a few severely thalassemic patients in our clinic for whom family tests have revealed compatible siblings. Soon after we de-tected our first patient who was a good candidate for a marrow transplant, Don Thomas reported the successful transplantation of a child with thalassemia. That result did not surprise us, given our successes with Wiskott-Aldrich syndrome. The question was not whether we *could* transplant patients with thalassemia. The ques-tion was whether we *should*.

Our view at the time was fairly simple. Patients, we believed, should be informed about the possibility of marrow transplanta-tion, and their families should be screened for a potential donor. Patients should be told exactly what the risk of death from the procedure or its failure was (50 percent or more in 1968), but that if they survived the treatment they would be free of transfusion and the risk of iron overload. Furthermore, they would be free of the enormous financial and emotional burden of our half-way measures. We also concluded that we should strongly urge patients to accept a transplant if they could not or would not comply with conservative treatment programs that now dramatically prolong life. This particularly applies to patients from less well developed countries where those treatments are more difficult to obtain or to children from parts of the United States where physicians may lack experience of the disease.

We still hold these opinions today about the role of marrow transplantation in the treatment of thalassemia. Data gathered in the United States and England show that the present risk of immediate death, graft failure, or profound disability from transplantation for thalassemia is now about 40 percent even in patients at or below the age of five. If we could believe that the risk of failure is much lower, we would urge *all* thalassemic patients with compatible donors to have a transplant as soon as the diagnosis is made.

In contrast to the experience in the United States, a marrow transplant center in Italy is reporting far better results in a very large clinical experience. They divide patients into different so-called prognostic groups and claim that about a tenth of their patients below the age of sixteen, those with low iron burden and little evidence of iron-induced tissue injury at the time of transplant, have a much better chance of survival. In this tiny subset, the risk of death or transplant failure is as low as 5 percent. Recently, a transplant center in Belgium has begun to transplant sickle cell anemia patients from Zaire (the former Belgian Congo). They report that they have transplanted more than twenty such patients and have cured 90 percent of them.

Not surprisingly, these recent results have caught the attention of hematologists around the globe. If inherited diseases of the marrow can be treated effectively with little or no risk, we have a new world before us. Yet there are cautionary notes. The experience in Italy and Belgium has not been replicated in this country, in Canada, or in England. Until it is, advice to patients must be guarded.

My own view of confusing results such as these is that the statistical likelihood of death and failure from marrow transplantation for nonmalignant bone marrow disease is about 25 percent in the United States and England. The results in the immune deficiencies are better. Transplant centers with poorer results are probably having a run of bad luck. Those that claim far better results may have a unique experience with a very small subset of patients. They may be dividing their patients into so-called prognostic groups that are poorly representative, cannot be broadly applied, and will not be reproducible in other centers. It is also possible that the patients treated in a particular center abroad may be more inbred than is the case in the United States and therefore may have less likelihood of developing graft-versus-host disease. For these reasons and others, the experience of one transplant center may not always be applicable to others, particularly if the centers are in different countries.

A few years ago, our pediatric oncology clinic had a very instructive experience. We did not have enough marrow transplant beds in our hospital to serve all of the patients with leukemia who were referred to us for the procedure. Therefore we sent many of our patients to another excellent and larger marrow transplant center that was managed by one of the graduates of our own hospital. We know him well, and we have complete confidence in his skill. That center was reporting spectacular results in marrow transplantation for leukemia, but our patients transplanted there did not do very well. The majority died of recurrent leukemia or graft-versus-host disease. There are several potential reasons for this apparent dichotomy. The center in question may have been reporting results in a selective way; for example, they may have been eliminating cases from inclusion in their reports that did not fit some artificial standard, and these may have been the very patients who fared poorly. On the other hand, the result may have simply represented a statistical fluke that would not be repeated in a subsequent series. There may have been something unique about the population of patients that we referred that made them more susceptible to failure. Finally, we may have failed to care for the patients adequately when they returned to our clinic for follow-up. All of these are possibilities, some more likely than others. No matter the reason(s), the stated results of one program's treatment may not be replicated in another group of patients.

Given all the uncertainties that affect interpretation of clinical data, how should a responsible physician or hospital advise patients, such as young children with thalassemia, who may have a matched sibling donor? My response remains based on fairly simple principles. I tell my patients that their present chance for success is about three out of four (much better than in 1968). I also tell them about the vastly better claims in Italy, but I warn them that the same results might not be reproducible and might not apply in their case. I then point out that the expected life span of a young thalassemic patient well managed with conservative therapy has improved. In the next decade there may be many developments in transplantation and even gene replacement therapy that could make a curative procedure less risky. However, conservative treatments demand slavish adherence to a disagreeable and very costly therapeutic program that depends on repeated blood transfusions that are themselves dangerous. I try to answer their many questions as carefully as I can, let them make up their own minds, and follow the course of their choice.

There are at least two critical points to emphasize about such medical Hobson's choices. The physician must be absolutely sure that he or she is following the therapeutic wishes of the parents and the patient. However, in such circumstances the physician must be very careful to be certain that the parents are actually making the best decision they can on behalf of their minor children and not on their own behalf. Here the physician runs very close to an unacceptable line of paternalism. In almost all cases, parents see a serious illness in one of their children through the eyes of the child and not merely through their own. But there are rare parents who are so anxious to rid themselves of a burden that they will unwittingly seize on a kill-or-cure therapy as the solution. In such cases, the child is a pawn rather than an object of parental devotion. The quality of the decision in such unusual circumstances needs to be examined very carefully, but the physician cannot take over the responsibility from the parents. This is why the circumstance skirts the line of paternalism and must be handled with great caution.

There is a second and even more sensitive issue. In pediatrics a decision to accept or reject a particular therapy is made by parents on behalf of a beloved child. If that decision has a bad outcome, the parents will be completely devastated by guilt. For that reason, the physician must find a way to make the parents believe that the decision, once made, is the one that he or she completely endorses. In other words, once the parents have expressed their wishes, the physician must lift the burden of responsibility from the shoulders of the parents and place it where it belongs, on his or her own back. But all this must be done without taking the choice away from the parents in the first place. The dialogue must be thorough enough to be sure of that result.

Present concerns about the quality of informed consent make that second duty very difficult to accomplish. Patients and their families are confronted with endless documents that detail every hazard of a procedure. The documents are read to them in ponderous tones, and they are filled with lugubrious paragraphs that begin with solemn phrases such as "I understand that . . ." Then the papers are signed in front of witnesses and filed with the hospital attorneys who created them under the tight supervision of the hospital's malpractice insurance carrier. This is no idle exercise. I regularly hear from broken-hearted parents whose children had transplants in other centers that they never knew the risks of the procedure. Often crying over the phone while they talk with me, they insist that they would never have permitted the treatment had they understood the hazards. Sometimes they want me to be a witness in a lawsuit against the center in which the transplant occurred, the suit based on insufficient quality of informed consent. When I ask my colleagues in those centers for a copy of the signed document, it is invariably careful and accurate.

The death of one's child is unbearable, and some parents who suffer this terrible loss can act irrationally. Hospitals, physicians, and their insurance carriers correctly conclude that they must be protected, particularly in the current climate of malpractice suits in the United States. Given all of this legal necessity, it is not easy to lift the burden from the shoulders of parents. But I always tell my residents and fellows that the role of the physician is to do the difficult at once, and to do the impossible tomorrow. There is no easy formula for how to go about this, but as Samuel A. Levine said to me in my internship year, "Worry about your patient. If you worry enough, you will do as good a job as you can."

Given all of these complex considerations, it is obvious that experimental medicine, particularly experimental therapeutics, requires an exact amalgam of experience, courage, compassion, and judgment. It is very hard to be certain that a high-risk procedure should be attempted in a given case. I can only say now, in retrospect, that I am glad that there was no compatible donor for Dayem. Our skills were not high enough at the time. Perhaps I wouldn't have taken the risk anyway, but I never had to test my judgment.

THE NEXT LETTER from Mrs. Saif was much less pleasing. "I am afraid this letter will not be as optimistic as the last. The reason is that on the thirty-first of October the doctor thought it was time for Dayem to be transfused. He had five grams of hemoglobin and he was still feeling great. So on the thirty-first he was transfused with 250 milliliters of washed cells. The next day his eyes were yellow and his face much darker—almost black, especially his forehead. The next day he was more or less normal but not at all with as much energy as he had with his first transfusion in Boston. Anyhow, two weeks later, his brother number two had the flu and a high fever. The next day Dayem came back from school very low, crying and with a terrible headache, so he said. I called the doctor and a blood test was done. He had only three grams of hemoglobin. He was hospitalized right away; he had a very strong cold with cough and fever. Dr. Herrera was very concerned about his heart condition so he called a cardiologist who didn't find anything alarming, but he advised the transfusion should be given very slowly. He was transfused with 300 milliliters in five days. The first transfusion raised the hemoglobin from 3.2 to 6.2. The second transfusion raised the hemoglobin from 6.2 to 6.9. The third transfusion was very difficult because the veins did not accept the blood, and finally, they found one of the foot veins, and the transfusion took place after six attempts. Now Dayem is in bed, he has his good humor back but he is still very weak and very

pale, and Dr. Herrera told me that many times a permanent transfusion is needed."

"I really am worried even knowing that Dr. Herrera is *the* pediatrician in Mexico so I have been told, but two transfusions in less
than two weeks (from the thirty-first until the fourteenth of November) left Dayem so weak even after the transfusions with a real
sick face. I think this is enough for an ignorant [sic] like me to be
worried. P.S. If after all that I have told you, you think that it's better
to bring Dayem to Boston, please tell me."

That letter immediately settled one important issue. Dayem
needed his spleen taken out right away.

The spleen is an organ the size of a flattened orange located
high in the left side of the abdomen. It is the most effective component of the body's scavenger mechanism. The rubbish-eating
cells called phagocytes ("eating cells") that line its narrow channels
cleanse the blood of unwanted particles such as bacteria and distorted cells. The splenic swamp is a challenge to normal red cells,
let alone injured thalassemic red cells. Dayem's abnormal red cells
had so stimulated the phagocytes (to use George Bernard Shaw's
phrase) in his spleen that the organ had become massively enlarged. Now those rubbish eaters were eating up normal transfused
cells as well as Dayem's abnormal ones. If we did not remove his
spleen, Dayem would require near-continuous transfusion. Furthermore, he might begin to make antibodies against transfused cells,
and such a catastrophe might make it impossible to transfuse him
at all.

I used cable, air mail, and phone to reach the family and Mickey
Herrera and to strongly recommend that Dayem return to Boston
immediately for removal of his spleen.

A few days later the family arrived, and Dayem was promptly
admitted for evaluation. The most striking observation was his
deep pigmentation, dark urine, and hugely distended belly. His
spleen was enormous, and his liver was enlarged as well. He was
simultaneously pale and jaundiced, and his heart was enlarged as
before. But there was no evidence of heart failure, and his hemoglobin was 6 grams per 100 milliliters, much better than the 1.5
grams per 100 milliliters with which we had begun.

We decided that we had a bit of time and elected to examine Dayem's splenic function more quantitatively. To do so, we carefully chose a compatible unit of red cells and labeled them with radioactive chromium before we infused them. The chromium was quite tightly bound to the red cells and provided a tag on the cells that we could follow in Dayem's body.

The chromium study confirmed our diagnosis. The labeled cells disappeared very rapidly from Dayem's circulation. Their life span was much shorter than would have been the case in a normal child. Furthermore, the radioactive chromium rapidly appeared in the spleen, as detected by a radioactivity monitor that we placed over his abdomen. This meant that Dayem's spleen was a major mischief-maker. It had been so stimulated by his misshapen cells that it was destroying all cells, even normal ones. That spleen had to come out.

In another meeting with Mrs. Saif, I explained the pros and cons of spleen removal in thalassemia. She had known since Dayem's first admission to our clinic that in children who had had years of stimulation of their spleens by their own abnormal red cells, removal of the spleen was almost always necessary to prevent rapid destruction of transfused red blood cells. In children started on transfusion at a very young age, the spleen often did not become large for many years, and in a few of these patients spleen removal could be avoided altogether. But sooner or later most children wound up having the operation in order for their bodies to make adequate use of the transfusions they had to have to stay alive.

But I had to re-emphasize that removal of the spleen is not without hazard. The spleen is the major filter of the circulation. Since it removes foreign particles, including bacteria, from the blood, spleenless children are at increased risk of dying from overwhelming bacterial infection. They, their families, and their pediatricians need to be aware of that risk, and broad spectrum antibiotics must be taken at the first sign of a serious infection. But it's not easy to distinguish an incipient serious bacterial infection from a trivial viral infection in the first few crucial hours or days. So patients must be trained to use good judgment and if necessary err on the side of taking antibiotics. Furthermore, patients must take a low dose of penicillin every day to prevent the appearance of pneumococcus bacteria in their blood. Pneumococcus is an airborne germ, and few of us fail to have it in cultures of our throats. But people with intact spleens rarely, if ever, allow that bug out of their throats and into their blood, where it can cause enormous mischief. It frequently enters the blood in those who contract pneumococcal pneumonia. That's a serious enough illness, but if caught early it can be treated very effectively with penicillin.

The hazard for a spleenless patient is that the organism can get into the blood, or even the spinal fluid, even when none of the classical symptoms of pneumonia are present. Such an episode begins with low-grade fever and muscle aches, a phase of the illness that is hard to distinguish from a viral flu-like illness. Then it explodes into meningitis, high fever, shock, and, frequently, fatal hemorrhage. There are some other bacteria that can behave in a similar fashion. The common *Hemophilus influenza* bacterium (not the virus) that until recently so often caused middle-ear infections and very serious bloodstream infections could occasionally cause a very similar problem in spleenless patients, as can, rarely, the even more common *Escherichia coli* that dominate our stools. Furthermore, these two organisms are not sensitive to penicillin. So to be on the safe side, the spleenless patient who might be getting such an infection must take a large dose of a broad spectrum antibiotic to ward off disaster.

Today we have effective vaccines that create antibodies against the pneumococcus and *H. influenza,* and we vaccinate our spleenless patients with these products to reduce the risk. But they must still take penicillin every day, and they are provided with broad spectrum antibiotics to take as soon as they get fever and muscle aches without the obvious cough and runny nose of a standard cold.

"On balance," I told Mrs. Saif, "removal of the spleen is still the best choice. It does carry the risk I just described, but without the operation his transfusion requirement will be too high. He will become iron overloaded so fast that we will lose him from iron toxicity within one or two years."

Mrs. Saif made the decision quickly. We would go ahead with the operation and be careful about subsequent infections. This was another example of high-risk medical decision-making. It had been a risk to transfuse him, but on balance the risk had to be taken. Now there was a risk associated with spleen removal. The operative risk was very low, but the post-operative risk would extend for the rest of his life. However, we could not successfully carry out the transfusion program without the operation. So we made the commitment and moved ahead.

The procedure was performed easily, though I worried about hemorrhage during the operation. The spleen had been hugely enlarged for so long that there might be very large veins and arteries supplying it with blood, and I was concerned that these could be torn during the surgery. But then, as now, Children's Hospital surgeons were particularly facile at removing spleens. They did the procedure frequently and were both speedy and accurate. Dayem was out of the operating room in an hour and sailed through the early days of recovery. I removed a small piece of the enormous spleen and examined it under the microscope. It was full of red cells so distorted by clumps of precipitated alpha chains that they were being destroyed by splenic rubbish eaters. The procedure had been absolutely necessary.

Shortly after the operation, we gave Dayem a substantial red cell transfusion, and to our enormous satisfaction and that of his mother, the transfused red cells survived. His hemoglobin rose to the normal range and stayed there for days. We had made the right decision. Dayem could return to Mexico and would do well.

A FEW DAYS after Dayem's discharge from the hospital, my wife and I invited him and his mother and brothers (who had accompanied him) to our house for a celebratory dinner. My school-aged children joined us, as did our less-than-brilliant dog. I watched nervously as Dayem made friends with that oafish but kind beast, which suddenly looked enormous to me. I was afraid he would jump on Dayem in his foolish fashion, throw him to the ground, and cause a fracture. The dog was promptly removed.

My oldest daughter, who was sixteen years old, was fascinated by Dayem. She has always loved little dolls, and Dayem, so tiny for his age yet with the intelligence and verbal skills of a six-year-old, was the most doll-like person she had ever seen. She couldn't take her eyes off him and his baby shoes except to cast a glance toward his mother. My daughter was smitten by Mrs. Saif, just as our staff had been. The combination of her handsome appearance and high intelligence, her humor and sophistication, made her an instant heroine in the eyes of an inexperienced American teenager trying to forge an identity, and I could see that Mrs. Saif had an instant affinity for my daughter. They became fast friends at first sight.

We set about to cook a perfect lamb dinner on the simple theory that all Arabs eat lamb at every meal. It was a concept we had gathered from watching films like *Four Feathers, Khartoum,* and *Lawrence of Arabia.* Our knowledge of the Arab world was pathetically thin and largely cinematic. That evening began our education.

Within moments we had launched into a discussion of the Israeli-Palestinian conflict, an issue that had preoccupied Mrs. Saif since her law school days in Damascus. Her innate sense of justice dominated her argument. She had complete respect for the plight of the Jewish victims of the Nazi holocaust and accepted the formation of the state of Israel, though her loyalties prevented her from expressing any support for a formal Jewish state. However, she passionately believed that the displaced Palestinians must have a homeland of their own, and it was not to be in either Lebanon, Jordan, or Syria. There was, in her view, enough blame for the plight of the Palestinians to be spread widely and thickly in the West, in the Arab world, in Israel, and among the Palestinians themselves. The issue before the world was to carve out a land that could become an Arab Palestinian state within the old borders of Palestine. No other solution would bring justice to the Middle East.

"Would that lead to peace and recognition of Israel's right to exist?" I asked.

"Intelligent people," she responded, "work out their differences when they respect each other's basic needs."

That conversation took place twenty-seven years ago. Mrs. Saif, my wife, and I have had many like it since, while the world still awaits that mutual recognition of basic needs. I naively believed then that if Mrs. Saif or someone like her could be put in sole charge of the Israeli-Palestinian conflict, it would be solved. But having watched the world behave in the decades since, I have become much more cynical. Few people would listen to a person who is so decent, intelligent, and fair. Even the martyrdom of Anwar Sadat and Count Folke Von Bernadotte have been to no avail. It is foolish to think that Mrs. Saif or any one person could find a simple solution to the mess in the Middle East, but the dream is worth savoring. And recently there has been a glimmer of hope.

The dinner over, and Dayem ready for a night's sleep, we said our farewells. I prepared a detailed letter to Mickey Herrera in which I described our patient's excellent response to removal of his spleen and advised him to continue the transfusion program that we had planned. We would remain in close contact. In a year we would repeat the x-rays of his bones and choose the next steps thereafter. I emphasized the importance of the daily dose of penicillin and told Mickey that we had advised Mrs. Saif to give Dayem oral antibiotics if she believed he had symptoms compatible with the early phases of a bloodstream bacterial infection. This would cause confusion for Mickey because he would be unable to confirm or rule out the diagnosis through a blood culture if Dayem had already taken a large dose of broad spectrum antibiotics. But we all agreed that in cases like this, it was better to err on the side of over-treatment.

Dayem returned to Mexico in mid-December 1968. I continued to think about him with great concern. Would he become infected? How rapidly would he develop iron overload? Would he have a fracture again before the transfusions could correct his bones? In early January of 1969, I wrote a note to his parents.

"Could you drop me a note about our boy. I am anxious to know how he is doing. No news is good news, but I believe there is an excellent Arab proverb which, translated, says, 'You better know what's going on.'"

A few days later a letter arrived from Mexico. "Dayem is feeling great and the last blood test was 8.6 grams and was 10 days ago. He is enjoying school, playing golf, and he is feeling very strong (he wants to fight, and run, and jump all the time)." The letter went on to describe how Dayem was handling his dependence on trans-fusions by using a mixture of television fantasy and his own fertile imagination. He was "Prince Planet" receiving energy from outer space in the form of transfusion, or he was the hero of *Run for Your Life*, a television series in which the central character is running from enemies who want his blood because it is so powerful. I was delighted with the letter and with all of the subsequent bulletins that came from Mexico.

In June of 1969 Dayem returned to Boston for reevaluation. He had been transfused every six to eight weeks, keeping his hemoglo-bin to between 8 and 11 grams per hundred milliliters of blood. We were terribly pleased when we saw him and wrote to Mickey Her-rera, "He has grown very well. In fact, his growth curves are ap-proaching a vertical axis."

When Dayem and his mother came again to our home for dinner on that third visit, my daughter could see that her doll was about to grow up. Though he was still very small for his age, he was clearly gaining height and weight and putting muscle on his bones. Even more gratifying was the pleasure that he took in his surround-ings. He seemed liberated, as though he knew that the fracture period was coming to an end.

Mrs. Saif reported that Dayem had been oddly inattentive at school, and his teachers wondered whether he actually heard them in the classroom. Our hearing and speech clinic confirmed that Dayem was partially deaf in both ears and that the difficulty was likely due to a defect in the tiny bones that transmit the sound from the eardrum to the auditory nerve. I wondered whether the enormous bone marrow growth he had experienced had stimulated abnormal bone marrow growth in those sound-transmitting bones, and whether this had somehow inhibited their function. If so, I reasoned, he should wear a hearing aid for a while and continue transfusion. As his long bones remodeled and became structurally sound, his tiny ear bones might also.

Six months later, in December of 1970, that theory was happily confirmed. New x-rays of Dayem's bones showed that they had greatly lengthened and had remodeled well. The cortex of the long bones—the part that forms the outer wall of the bone cylinder and provides the supporting structure—had markedly thickened. The marrow space had receded. Dayem now had nearly normal bones, and for the first time he was free of the risk of fracture following trivial accidents. Furthermore, his hearing was nearly normal, presumably because marrow cells had retreated from his middle ear bones. He could get rid of the hearing aid. We were clearly moving in the right direction.

By the spring of 1971 Dayem, now nine years old, was doing beautifully. He kept up with his classmates in all activities, was growing like a weed, assumed his rightful place as the leader of his younger brothers, and was a joy in every way but one. The exception was his face. The flat facial bones do not remodel following transfusion of patients with thalassemia. Once the distortion occurs, it cannot be reversed. The large bones and even, as we learned from Dayem, the ossicles of the ear can respond, but the face remains distorted in a gargoylesque fashion. One teenaged patient whom I saw in consultation had such a misshapen face that she refused to leave her house except at night because she was so fearful of being taunted. Since Dayem was now only nine years old, he did not yet notice the severity of his deformity, but I feared for that moment. I thought it would inevitably come, particularly as he approached the self-conscious teenage years when appearance seems to matter more than anything else. For the moment, however, all was well.

His mother wrote in May of 1971 that she had seen Professor Fanconi and had brought him up to date on Dayem's progress. Always the thoughtful gentleman, Fanconi expressed his pleasure at Dayem's well-being, and did not remind her that her joy would be short-lived if we did not find a way to eliminate the iron that was steadily accumulating in Dayem's body.

Iron Overload

A T   T H E   E N D   O F   1 9 7 1, when Dayem was nine and a half years old, he was continuing his very satisfactory growth. He would be smaller than most boys his age, but he was growing, and his bones and muscles were in excellent condition. School progress was satisfactory. His face remained distorted, but his heart function was generally normal. There were, however, two ominous findings. His skin was bronzed, and his liver was enlarged. Both are manifestations of iron overload.

One year later at the next check-up, Dayem's skin was even darker, and the iron content of his blood had risen to a very high level. Indeed, all of his body's special iron-binding plasma protein (called transferrin) was completely saturated with iron, and careful measurements suggested that iron was spilling into other proteins as well. Our hands were being forced. We would have to find a way to reduce his iron overload.

Iron overload and iron toxicity from chronic red cell transfusion are major threats to all patients with transfusion-dependent thalassemia and to any other patient who requires repeated red cell transfusion over a long time period. Death is inevitable if the iron is not removed. There was no hope for any solution until John Nielands, a member of the Biochemistry Department at the University of California in Berkeley, began to ask a fundamental question. How do bacteria, which absolutely require iron for their growth, extract it from the soil in which they live? Nielands found that bacteria synthesize several different compounds that have a remarkably high and very selective affinity for iron. When iron enters the bacterial cell wall, one of these compounds, which Nielands called a siderophore (from the Greek *sideros,* iron, and *phoros,* bearing or carrying) grabs it and holds it in the cell, giving it up only to the enzymes that require it.

Siderophores are members of a class of chemicals called chelators (from the Greek *chele,* claw). These compounds are capable of binding metals or other substances with very high affinity. They may bind a metal in the body so tightly that they never give it up; rather, the chelators are excreted in the urine or stool still carrying their prey. Hence, they can be very useful in treating people for lead, copper, or iron poisoning.

Nielands was not interested in the therapy of human disease. He was instead fascinated by the methods by which bacteria deal with their environment. Having read of Nielands's work, Swiss academic scientists in collaboration with researchers at the Ciba-Geigy Pharmaceutical Company in Basel decided to try to find a clinically useful siderophore in various species of fungi that were being examined by Ciba-Geigy for possible antibiotics. Given the enormous range of compounds that primitive organisms like bacteria and fungi produce, it is perhaps not surprising that the researchers found an interesting substance which, when bound to iron, turned from colorless to a lovely shade of red. Since the compound has several oxygen molecules linked to amine groups (amines are nitrogen molecules to which hydrogen is attached), the compound was called ferroxamine. The colorless iron-free derivative compound was named deferroxamine and later given the trade name Desferal. Heinrich Keberle, a chemist at Ciba-Geigy, set about to develop both of them.

Though Keberle was a basic scientist like Nielands, he worked for a pharmaceutical company, and he immediately began to wonder whether ferroxamine would be a useful drug in the treatment of iron deficiency. Iron deficiency is one of the commonest diseases among humans. Millions suffer from it, particularly women with heavy menstrual flow. The treatment is simple: iron salts. But iron salts often irritate the gastrointestinal tract and can cause constipation and bloating. Patients sometimes dislike the treatments intensely. In the 1960s when Keberle was working on ferroxamine, he hoped that it would deliver iron to the blood without irritating the gastrointestinal tract. The deferroxamine that resulted from the iron delivery would be excreted in the urine.

Keberle was soon to be disappointed. Neither ferroxamine nor deferroxamine were absorbed from the intestine. But Keberle noted that when deferroxamine was given by mouth, it came out in the stool as ferroxamine, having sought out and bound the iron that was in the intestine. That gave him another idea. He injected deferroxamine into iron-loaded animals. To his delight, a large amount of ferroxamine appeared in the urine. In fact, the urine turned red, it was so laden with iron. Keberle did not have a drug that would be useful in iron deficiency, but he might have a chelation approach to iron overload.

Clinical trials with Desferal promptly began in Switzerland, and they were somewhat encouraging. The drug was not absorbed from the intestine, but a single intramuscular injection of half a gram to a chronically transfused patient would lead to the release of up to five milligrams of iron in the urine. Since there is one milligram of iron in one milliliter of red cells, a daily dose of half a gram (500 milligrams) of Desferal for one month would lead to the loss of the amount of iron contained in a little less than one unit (200 milliliters or a half pint) of red cells.

Since patients with thalassemia receive considerably more than one unit of red cells per month, it was clear that one could never achieve a state of negative iron balance with this drug at that dose and by that route of administration. So the Swiss physicians treated some patients with three injections of intramuscular Desferal a day. That worked. Some of the patients lost as much as 15 milligrams of iron a day. If that rate of loss continued for years, it would eventually lead to depletion of the large stores of iron they had accumulated.

Keberle and the Swiss physicians presented their results at a meeting of the International Society of Hematology in Mexico City in 1968. The audience was transfixed. Here was the first effective treatment of iron overload. Lost sight of was the fact that the stoical patients had to endure three painful intramuscular injections every day. Desferal is quite irritating to muscle, and very few adults would be willing to be subjected to this level of pain on a routine basis. A three-injection daily routine would be out of the question for children. No child could tolerate it.

It did not take long for the Mexico City audience to learn the reality of intramuscular Desferal. One dose per day was all that most patients could take, and a single dose was not enough. After a brief flurry of interest, Desferal was largely abandoned, but unknown to Keberle and his colleagues, the Desferal story was just beginning.

South African physicians are well acquainted with iron overload. Many Africans make a beer that is brewed at home in iron pots. The content of iron in the beer is enormous, and a high proportion of black Africans seem to have a genetic characteristic that permits them to absorb much more iron from the intestine than do normal individuals. The result is frequently severe iron overload, with its attendant heart failure, liver dysfunction, bronze skin, and diabetes from damage to the pancreas.

In addition to these effects, iron overload decreases the body's stores of vitamin C, and vitamin C makes iron more available for chelation. This finding influenced several groups in England and the United States to give vitamin C (ascorbic acid) to iron-overloaded patients just before Desferal was injected. Most patients excreted even more iron when they took the vitamin.

At the end of 1972—when Dayem was ten years old—I put him on a program of a single intramuscular Desferal injection three times a week, with supplementary vitamin C. The painful injections were given by Mrs. Saif, and Dayem disliked them intensely, but he took them because he had no choice. Overall, the results were disappointing. He excreted three times as much iron when a large dose of vitamin C was taken before each injection, but his iron excretion was never very impressive. I maintained the program only because I had nothing else to offer, but I was not at all hopeful that I was doing him very much good.

In an effort to increase his excretion, I asked him to take the Desferal shots every day. Again, he did it because he had no choice.

His mother faithfully administered the injections, though she hated giving them as much as he loathed receiving them.

In 1974 Dayem, now twelve years old, left Mexico with his family to live in London, where his father would represent his company's interests in Europe. Dayem was to remain in England for five years until he was seventeen, supervised closely by our colleagues in London. He returned to us for annual check-ups.

During that five-year period I decided that if he and others were to be saved, I would have to wage a pincer attack on thalassemia. I would need to improve our chelation strategy, and at the same time my colleagues and I would need to uncover the molecular basis of the disease so that a fundamental and lasting treatment could be developed. Time was of the essence. The results of transfusion had helped our patients, including Dayem, to grow and develop, but several of them were beginning to suffer from the ravages of iron overload. Heart failure, diabetes, and liver failure were becoming rampant. Intramuscular Desferal was accomplishing very little with or without vitamin C. We would lose them all if we did not act swiftly.

As I glumly reviewed the results in the mid-1970s, it became obvious to me that the problem with Desferal was the route of administration of the drug, not the drug itself. Patients can take grams of Desferal daily for years, with little or no toxicity. Its action is very specific for iron. The problem, I realized, is *how* we give it. If we could give it continuously instead of as a single injection in the muscle, I believed that much more iron would be excreted.

Accordingly, Richard Propper (one of my fellows who later become associated with several biotechnical companies), Susan Shurin (currently chief of pediatric hematology at Case Western Reserve University), and I planned some simple experiments. We would give one of our patients a dose of Desferal by continuous intravenous drip and compare its effect on iron excretion to the standard intramuscular injection. The results that we described in 1976 when Dayem was fourteen years old were remarkable. The patient excreted a vast amount of iron while the drug was administered by vein slowly and continuously because each molecule of the drug had a greater opportunity to encounter an iron molecule during the continuous dosing. At the doses we used, we would clearly achieve negative iron balance in our patients and presumably reverse the consequences of iron overload.

But our enthusiasm was tempered by a practical problem. How could we give the drug continuously? Obviously it would be impossible for patients to administer the drug to themselves by intravenous drip all day, every day. What young person could carry around a bottle on an IV pole for the rest of her life, even assuming that we could gain continuous access to a peripheral vein? So the idea, though excellent in many respects, was useless without a practical solution to the delivery problem. Richard Propper suddenly had a very good idea. He decided to determine whether the drug would be continuously absorbed if we injected it slowly into the fat pads just under the skin—a subcutaneous delivery. In preliminary tests conducted in 1977, the subcutaneous route worked very well. Large amounts of iron were excreted. We could easily achieve negative iron balance, and we calculated that with three or four years of treatment or even less, we would rid the patients of most of the iron that had been accumulated from years of transfusion.

But how would we deliver the drug continuously under the skin? No one would expect parents to give their children four or five subcutaneous injections every day. It's difficult enough to give severe diabetics two subcutaneous injections of insulin a day. To deal with that issue, Richard decided to have a small pump built that could be battery operated and slowly inject Desferal through a needle placed under the skin. The patient's parents would simply place the needle subcutaneously and attach the tubing to the pump. The pump would be so light that it could be worn on the child's belt in a holster.

The idea was so simple that we felt like kicking ourselves for not considering it much earlier. Soon we were off seeking a pump maker and found a bright young entrepreneur who had a machine shop in his basement in Brooklyn. The prototype pumps were considerably larger than we liked; the children looked like cowboys carrying Colt revolvers, and many were embarrassed at the thought of wearing the pumps to school. But the system worked well for most of our patients. Just as we had predicted from the preliminary studies, they excreted large amounts of iron every day.

The development of the subcutaneous infusion pump has had a much broader application than in thalassemia alone. The idea was snapped up by oncologists, who use it today for the delivery of certain cancer drugs. And clinical researchers focusing on diabetes are working on subcutaneous infusion pumps to deliver insulin to patients with certain forms of the disease that are particularly difficult to control. It often turns out to be the case in medical research that investigators focusing on a particular problem invent an approach that can be widely used by others focusing on different disorders.

BUT THERE WERE PROBLEMS with our new approach to dealing with iron overload. There are always problems when difficult diseases must be managed by halfway measures that ameliorate symptoms and complications but do not cure. First of all, while vitamin C supplements did enhance iron excretion, they also increased iron absorption from the intestine and were implicated in the sudden onset of heart failure in some patients. There was no clear proof of that dangerous effect, but there was circumstantial evidence, so we decided to eliminate the vitamin C supplementation.

The second issue was skin irritation. Though many if not most of the patients tolerated the subcutaneous administration of Desferal, some did not. They developed hot and painful or itchy sores at the site of injection. In most of the patients the reaction was abolished if we added a tiny amount of a cortisone-like drug to the Desferal.

But the most intractable difficulty arose from the substantial resistance to the whole plan by our patients. And in fairness, they did have problems with the contraption. There were daily battles between mothers and young children when the needle had to be changed. School-age children resented wearing the bulky pump in a holster on their belts, and they hated having to place the needle under the skin of their abdomen and thread the plastic tubing out through their clothes and into the pump. The biggest problems arose with adolescents. Teenagers—particularly teenaged girls, whose dread of looking different often overcomes any other fear— found the rig unacceptable. It was a constant reminder of their illness, and emphasized the difference between them and their friends. When they put it on, they could smell their own mortality, and they hated it. The fact that their urine was red all the time because they were eliminating so much iron thrilled their doctors, but it disgusted them.

Pleased with what we had created, and having published the new concept in leading journals, we found ourselves exhorting our young patients to be sensible and adjust to our marvelous idea. It *was* marvelous, but several didn't think so. Some went on strike and refused to wear the pump. Others said they would, but we knew they were cheating. I began to wonder what Dayem's reaction to the new Desferal plan would be. He would be due for his annual check-up in a little more than a month. Would he cooperate, or would he try to avoid the whole thing? He was growing up, and he was living in a teenage fast lane in London. I had my doubts that he would be a model patient.

Cooperation with the new treatment plan would prove to be one of the most difficult issues that I would have to face in my research career. Some important help came from my Oxford University colleagues, who showed that an overnight subcutaneous infusion of Desferal would induce almost as much iron excretion as a 24-hour infusion. That was a boon, particularly to children and teenagers who could be free of the annoying and very visible pump during school. But unbeknownst to us at the time, the idea created yet another difficulty.

Iron overload is an insidious problem. Most of the excess iron is locked in a huge storage pool contained within rubbish-collecting cells and in membrane-encircled lumps in other cells, where it cannot do any direct damage. Only a small amount is actually free in cells to electrocute normal tissues, but that small free pool is continuously replenished from the storage pool. In our initial use of the Desferal pump in patients with heart failure, we noticed that when they received 24-hour infusion, they recovered from heart failure far faster than could be accounted for by their excretion of iron. Clearly, the constant Desferal infusion must have immediately chelated the small but particularly toxic iron pool in the heart (as well as in the liver and pancreas) and driven it into the stools and urine. During round-the-clock treatment, the huge storage pool slowly would empty into the smaller pool, where the Desferal would capture it. But if for half the day patients did not receive any Desferal, the small toxic pool in the tissues would be fed from the larger storage pool, and this build-up of iron in the heart, liver, and pancreas cells during the rest period would continue to electrocute those organs. This damage was done despite the fact that these patients were excreting almost as much iron as those on 24-hour treatment.

That rather subtle scenario did not occur to us at the time that the group at Oxford made their contribution. We were concentrating then on how we might be able to persuade our patients to accept the program at all, and the overnight infusion proposal was much more attractive to most of the patients than was our all-day and all-night treatment. So I decided to use it.

Ten years later, in 1985, my colleagues and I were able to report spectacular results for patients who were put on a five-nights-a-week schedule at an early age, before irreversible tissue damage had occurred, and who cooperated with the treatment. Very young preschool patients cooperated well because their parents forced it on them, and their morale was high because they did not have a distorted face. Those who were treated very early in life with transfusion continued to look almost normal, and they were physically fit. Many of the children who began on subcutaneous Desferal before the age of ten are now old enough to have contracted heart disease, but few if any of them have done so. In fact, over 90 percent are free of heart disease after fourteen years of follow-up. Accordingly, their attitude is very positive, and they have tended to remain on the program even during their teenage and young adult years.

Later, we discovered that the age at which treatment is begun is not the critical factor. Patients who started the nighttime program before any tissue damage had occurred, and who adhered tightly to the treatment schedule and maintained low burdens of iron, remained free of heart disease in their teenage years, regardless of the age at which they started treatment.

But patients who began nighttime Desferal after iron stores were already elevated and heart damage had occurred, or who failed to adhere closely to the treatment program, did poorly. A substantial fraction have developed heart disease. Many were not transfused until they had already developed irreversible facial changes, and they suffered from poor self-esteem, which in turn undermined their compliance with the program.

It was terribly painful for us to watch several adolescents who we had treated for many years begin to develop heart disease and die. They had been the subjects of the initial clinical research on Desferal, and we had worked out all of the principles of the treatment program by studying their responses to different doses of the drug, routes of administration, and schedules. They had been willing to spend weeks in the hospital in our clinical research center, patiently collecting their urine and stools while we performed iron-balance studies that tested the efficacy of one regimen or another. We had encouraged them to believe that our approach to Desferal treatment, particularly the use of subcutaneous infusion with the newly developed pumps on a five-night-a-week schedule, would be successful. We felt confident that they could have a healthy future if they would comply with the program as we defined it.

One after another, many of these brave young people—whose iron stores had been ruinously high for years before the Desferal program had been conceived—developed heart failure, and a large fraction of them died. The tragedy of their illness and inexorable death horrified the survivors. What good was all this attention to the details of transfusion and this slavish adherence to a daily encounter with Desferal if the ultimate result was to be a slow death from heart failure?

We were very frustrated. We had developed an effective therapy, but—we now knew from these tragic deaths—only for those who had no organ damage when treatment began and who were faithful in carrying out the program. The overnight infusion scheme, while more acceptable to patients, was not a safe approach for those who already had established organ damage from iron overload. For them, only treatment around the clock with Desferal could protect them from heart failure.

Many of our adolescent and young adult patients, seeing the death of their peers, believed that they were going to die no matter what they did, and they saw that we seemed helpless to prevent the inevitable. They began to refuse to take the subcutaneous injections. They complained bitterly about the pumps. They hated to go out in the evening with a pump held to a strap around their waist, and most refused to go to school with one. They insisted on a weekend off from the rig and would not hear of a seven-day, all-day schedule. They simply didn't believe that the extra commitment would help them when the five-night-a-week schedule would not. We knew of course how they felt. How can you make love with a pump on your hip attached to a needle in your stomach? What does a girl think when she puts her arm around your waist and feels a pump under your jacket?

It was obvious, we thought, that we needed a different kind of chelator—not a new pump but a new drug, one that could be taken by mouth, was absorbed readily in the stomach or the intestines, was retained for a reasonable time in the plasma, was capable of entering cells and chelating iron, and was capable as well of exiting the cells laden with iron on the way to excretion in the urine. Fortunately, we were not alone in the quest. Colleagues in Cleveland, New York, Gainesville, Jerusalem, and London were hard at work on the problem, but we knew that there would never be any significant success unless a major drug company took an interest.

As we reviewed the drug companies and their commitments, it became very obvious that only one of them, Ciba-Geigy in Basel, would have any reason to be interested in developing an oral iron chelator. Unfortunately, even their interest would prove to be limited. Though there are thousands of patients with thalassemia, indeed a few million in the world, most are in underdeveloped countries where the health budgets are very low. Desferal is prohibitively expensive in those countries. Ciba-Geigy had already invested heavily in Desferal. Sales of a new drug would not be high enough to justify the enormous development costs that would be incurred. In fact, a few years before, Ciba-Geigy had almost pulled Desferal off the market, arguing that its sales did not justify the cost of its production. The entire community of physicians interested in the disease protested that decision and persuaded the company to change its attitude. With all of that background, the chances for the development of a new orally active iron chelator seemed very bleak.

There was another reason for gloom as well. It was hard to believe that anyone would be lucky enough to create a drug that was as nontoxic as Desferal. After all, patients had to take almost two grams of the drug every day for a lifetime. There are very few drugs that can be taken at that dose and for that length of time without serious complications. Even aspirin would be likely to exhibit serious toxicity at that dose taken for many years. Why, we wondered, would a company invest in a new drug when the outlook for success is bleak, and when an adequate if less than ideal compound is already in hand?

Nothing ventured, nothing gained. I traveled to Basel to visit with the Ciba-Geigy scientists to see what ideas they might have about an orally active substitute for Desferal. There I was introduced to Heinrich Keberle himself, the Ciba scientist who had first studied Desferal after its discovery in an extract of a fungus and had been responsible for bringing it to market. Now he had risen to become a top executive in the company, and naturally I expected him to be deeply interested in the chelation problem. I was disappointed. As a senior executive, he had become a typically conservative guardian of the company's assets. He told me bluntly that Ciba-Geigy had done all it could or should do in the iron chelator field. There was not enough reason to make the investment that would be required to find another drug.

Fortunately, Keberle, though highly respected, was not joined in his opinion by all of the members of the Ciba-Geigy elite. The company gave me a very careful and sympathetic hearing and turned me over to Heinrich Peter, one of their highly skilled synthetic chemists. Peter is an expert on the chemistry of chelators, and he was fascinated by the complexity of synthesis that would be required if an orally active, nontoxic drug was to be produced.

In fact, he had been quietly working on the problem for some time and confided to me that he had actually prepared a few compounds that looked interesting. One or two had already been screened in rodents, but they needed to be examined carefully in monkeys because gastrointestinal function in rodents is unique and does not tell us much about how the drug would be absorbed in humans. Primates, though much more expensive, are the only satisfactory models of human absorption and toxicity.

Though Ciba-Geigy officialdom had been willing to look the other way when Peter went through some synthetic gymnastics, made some interesting compounds, and tested them in a few rats, they were not willing to invest in a more elaborate primate colony. If Peter wished to explore his compounds further, he would have to find another way.

I ALWAYS ENJOY watching how a huge bureaucracy like an international drug company finds a way to bend a policy. They were certainly not going to permit Peter to establish a large iron chelator research program in-house—not when someone with the international prestige of Heinrich Keberle was opposed to it. But Ciba-Geigy and other large multinationals do have grant-in-aid programs for the support of research in universities and hospitals. Those grant programs are now growing very rapidly as the companies realize that they can often gather useful information faster and more efficiently by giving support to independent scientists. This, they reckon, shortens their own payrolls and lowers their overhead by reducing the fringe benefits they would have to pay to their own employees and by decreasing the need for office and laboratory space. Furthermore, they can shop around widely for the precise skills they need to do a specific piece of research, and they can keep their commitments relatively short term, dropping what doesn't work and capitalizing on what does. As a result, grants from drug and biotechnical companies are becoming increasingly significant parts of university and teaching hospital research budgets. There are problems of course, as there always are when drug companies interact with universities.

The first sensitive issue arises from the basic differences in the missions of commercial enterprises and universities. Companies are interested in patents and profits. Universities are supposed to be interested in the free exchange of ideas. Recently, however, universities have been taking an increasing interest in patents and profits because the cost of doing research is in an ever-rising spiral. Grants alone will not pay the freight. So the universities and research-oriented hospitals are loosening their monastic devotion to a free exchange of ideas and have started keeping secrets until their patent attorneys tell them that it's safe to talk.

However, the universities and research hospitals do not want to accept money from a company that has too many strings of silence attached. A compromise has to be reached, and it usually is attained by establishing firm guidelines on publication. Companies that make grants to universities and research hospitals do receive advance warning of pending publication and are given time to deal with legal issues, but the time is strictly limited.

Recently Congress has become interested in the arrangements between universities and commercial companies, particularly foreign ones. Why, certain congressmen ask, should foreign companies capitalize on research done at U.S. taxpayer expense in American universities? That debate could get very serious, and it might get nasty. In fact, one research institute has already been forced by congressional pressure to alter a relationship with a Swiss pharmaceutical company when that particular arrangement was found wanting by a vociferous congressional critic.

A second area of tension is about research overhead, or what is known among the experts as the indirect costs of doing research. Most of us understand that research is carried out by scientists who must be paid and who incur costs because they buy supplies and equipment and hire technicians, postdoctoral fellows, and secretaries to perform and describe their experiments. These are the direct costs of doing research. But many outsiders and even many insiders do not sufficiently appreciate the costs involved in heating and lighting a research building, establishing a research library, running cafeterias to feed the scientists, providing them with security, guarding their animal colonies against vandalism by animal rights zealots, making sure that human subjects are treated with exquisite care, hiring attorneys to review protocols for informed consent and to defend the institution, when necessary, from litigation, or remodeling and rebuilding a research facility to meet the demands of new technology. All of these are indirect costs—they are extremely high and are bitterly disputed today.

For years, only the federal government has been willing to pay its full and fair share of the indirect costs of research programs sponsored by the National Institutes of Health, the National Science Foundation, and other government agencies. Private foundations such as the American Heart Association and the American Cancer Society have been unwilling to do so and so have most drug companies. But universities, and particularly their research-oriented faculty members, cannot support their laboratories with federal grants alone. They fight hard for and eagerly accept grants for direct costs from private foundations and companies, yet the end result is a large deficit in the indirect-cost budgets of the universities and hospitals. This has influenced the universities and hospitals to try to get as much indirect-cost support as possible from the federal government. Universities, research institutes, and hospitals hire as many gimlet-eyed, green-shaded accountants as they can afford. The task of this army in the business office is to pore over all of the federal indirect-cost regulations and get as much money into the indirect-cost till as they possibly can. Some universities, including my own, have become absolute experts at the indirect-cost game, but at the end of the year they still lose massive amounts of money doing research.

Recently one or two congressmen have decided to demonize the universities over the indirect-cost issue. The reasons for some of their actions are not entirely clear. To give them their due, they are correctly worried that the indirect-cost fraction of the federal biomedical research budget is getting out of hand. This is occurring in part because grant-givers other than the federal government do not pay their fair share; in part because the indirect costs have risen as new technologies have been developed; and in large part because the federal government has made a decision to assign the cost of new and remodeled research facilities to the indirect-cost fraction of individual research grants instead of creating a separate competitive program to which research-oriented institutions could apply for funds to help them build new facilities. Since the cost of construction is buried in the indirect-cost fraction of the research grants themselves, institutions whose researchers are high achievers in the federal grant competition have embarked on massive new building programs. The buildings are erected with borrowed money, and the interest payments are assigned as indirect costs to the federal grants. Since this sort of game is the only one in town, one university or hospital after another has engaged in bidding wars for competitive scientists and then embarked on expansion programs built on the indirect-cost money that they hope to extract from the federal grants those scientists land. Furthermore, institutions that have never before had a large commitment to research have joined the game because it seems to be an easy way to acquire new science facilities.

This Ponzi-like scheme is particularly dangerous for the universities and hospitals because it depends on an ever-increasing federal biomedical research budget. That budget has in fact been accelerating at a dramatic pace over the years. But as was true of the original Ponzi scheme, the bubble is bursting. The federal biomedical research budget is not going to accelerate at the rate that it has been growing in recent years. In fact, it is now declining in constant dollars. This is because there is nothing in the modern world as wasteful and hideously mismanaged as the health care budget of the United States. The management of the United Nations looks like a model of efficiency compared with the nightmare of our national health care system. The American biomedical research budget competes within our failed health program with milk for babies, vaccinations, care of the aged, and all of the other costs that a decent society incurs. In a nation that allows (indeed, encourages) the delivery of basic and specialized health care to be completely out of control, that has 30 or 40 million citizens who are uninsured, and that is operating with a terrifying overall budget deficit, it is little wonder that the very small fraction of the health and human services budget devoted to biomedical research (about one percent) is endangered.

The above-mentioned congressmen, who have proposed no useful resolution of the problem, have decided instead to scapegoat the universities and hospitals. It is always comforting and politically safe to find a villain, and universities and big hospitals are attractive targets because they appear rich and elite and do not pay taxes on most of their land and buildings. Furthermore, they are filled with tenured faculty members who are not afraid to thumb their noses at congressmen. Unfortunately, however, these same congressmen have found some examples of mismanagement of indirect costs within a few of the larger and very visible universities. Therefore, they have loudly shouted that our failure to control indirect costs lies not in our system but in the venal acts of the universities themselves.

There have, in fact, been some poor accounting practices and some less than acceptable interpretations of reimbursement rules by some universities. They need to be, and they are being, corrected. But the amounts of money involved have been tiny. The huge drain of indirect costs on the research grant budget continues because we have actually over-built our research facilities, just as we have over-built our health care facilities. We will not get our biomedical research and health care budgets in line until we refocus both systems, and no university nor any hospital will be the first to volunteer to go away. In fact, we desperately need to plan our health care and health research programs, decide upon their appropriate size and scope, and properly budget for those that must be retained in the national interest. That will require effective leaders in the federal government and the private sector who enjoy near-impossible tasks and who do not pander to every pressure group, including my own.

The third issue that affects relationships between for-profit companies and universities is the participation of faculty members (particularly research-oriented, hospital-based faculty) in commercially sponsored research. Some of the most important inventions that have emerged from the molecular revolution in biology have come from the hands of university and hospital faculty. Many of these inventions have led to therapeutic drugs that can earn many millions for companies that produce them and for their stockholders. This creates a serious ethical dilemma, particularly for physicians, but for basic scientists as well.

A physician has only one viable relationship to a patient. The physician is the servant of the patient. The physician's sole interest in that relationship must be the patient's welfare. There cannot be the slightest hint of a hidden agenda in the physician-patient nexus. This does not, of course, mean that the physician is the patient's slave. The physician or the physician's clinic should usually charge for the physician's services unless the patient is destitute. But the therapeutic or diagnostic procedures that are advised by the physician must not carry a secondary gain for the physician. If the physician is an inventor of a product and derives royalties from its use, is a significant stockholder in the company that sells it, or if he collects consultant fees from that company, neither the physician nor anyone in the line of the physician's authority or influence should have anything to do with the administration of the product to patients in research trials.

Many of my colleagues in the basic sciences believe that the same considerations apply to basic science professors who train graduate students or post-doctoral fellows in their laboratories. Those students and fellows come to the laboratories in good faith that their professor will guide them in experiments that are the best for science and not necessarily the best for the professor's pocketbook. Professors should not own stock in or collect royalties or fees from companies that make products that they use or examine in their laboratories.

Though I believe very strongly in these broad rules of behavior, many companies and some faculty members take a different position. The dissenting companies hold that it is important to have fiscal relationships with the individuals with whom they work, believing that those who have a financial stake in an enterprise will be loyal to it and more effective. They also believe that personal financial incentives are necessary to maintain a vigorous climate of invention.

Clearly, we have to define a compromise between these two positions, and I believe that we have found a reasonable if not perfect one at Harvard. Companies should continue to support the research activities of faculty members, but they should pay their royalties or consultant fees and stock contributions to the faculty member's institution rather than to the faculty member as an individual. The institution should treat these monies just like any other research grant. The funds should be used to support the academic effort or even the salary of the faculty member and his or her staff. In that way, the faculty member can pursue whatever line of research is of interest without having a personal financial stake in the outcome.

The compromise is not ideal. No compromise covers every contingency, but it does prevent the physician or the basic scientist from realizing an unsavory secondary gain, and at the same time it promotes entrepreneurial research. It does, however, place the institution in the position of gaining financially from research carried out on patients for whom the institution is responsible. That is a subtle but important problem that requires further studies. We need experience with this compromise, and we will surely get it during the next few years.

WHEN the Ciba-Geigy officials finally decided to support Peter's search for an oral iron chelator, they elected to award us a small research grant to establish an experimental model of iron chelation in an iron-overloaded primate. We worked with expert colleagues at the University of Lowell in Lowell, Massachusetts, who specialize in nutritional studies in primates, and began the difficult task of establishing iron balance studies in those animals. When the animals were well trained, they were injected with large amounts of iron and then received either intramuscular or oral Desferal, or an intramuscular or an oral dose of one of Peter's new chelators.

We were very excited when the first results showed that an oral dose of one of the new drugs was extremely effective. Whereas oral Desferal had, as expected, no effect on iron elimination, the new drug promptly and efficiently removed large amounts of iron from the overloaded animals.

Now we had a drug that could remove iron when given by mouth, but we had no idea of its safety. Indeed, there was preliminary evidence in the rodent studies that the drug might damage the kidneys. We had no capacity to do toxicity studies; that is a specialty of its own. Ciba-Geigy would not do the studies either, because they had no commitment to the development of the drug.

We were completely hamstrung until the National Institutes of Diabetes, Digestive and Kidney Diseases, which had responsibility within NIH to find a better chelator for chronically transfused patients, stepped in and agreed to support toxicity studies in rats with a contract awarded to a toxicology laboratory in New York. Sadly, the new drug proved to be toxic particularly to the kidneys. But that did not discourage Peter. He went on to synthesize several modifications of the compound and established a much larger primate evaluation program with our colleagues in Gainesville, Florida, who could devote far more resources to the model and were expert in its management. Their most recent results are encouraging. They have evaluated compounds prepared by Peter that are very active in iron-overloaded primates, and one of them is both highly effective and appears (on initial evaluation) to be much less toxic. Long-term toxicity studies, now in progress, are beginning to cause concern, however.

Other classes of drugs have been studied in Jerusalem, New York, and Cleveland. They are not nearly as active as the new Ciba-Geigy drugs, and they have not yet been subjected to detailed toxicity studies, but the work demonstrates that there are distinct possibilities for improvement upon the present Desferal regimen.

The group in London at the University College Hospital has come up with some very interesting findings. They have studied an entirely different class of compounds called the pyridones, again with the recent support of Heinrich Peter. One compound was rather unwisely rushed into human trials by an individual who had worked with the group at University College Hospital and then left for another hospital, where he gave the drug to patients without the permission of his former colleagues. This, understandably, led to bad blood between the two groups.

Medical research can have its ugly side. It is a competitive affair, as it should be. Competition, the desire to get there first, the hopes for adulation, for prizes, for promotion—these are vital ingredients in a national or international research program. When young people enter a research career and choose role models, they usually pick successful investigators who have discovered something important and are gaining the rewards of discovery. Only a competitive system will maintain such models and induce young people to make the sacrifices in time and effort that they must make if anything of value is to emerge from the laboratory.

Competition has to have rules of behavior, however. There is a very important code of ethics in science, built on trust and confidence in colleagues, that cannot be violated. If a scientist is untruthful in a publication or in a presentation; if data are deliberately mishandled or presented fraudulently; or if the essential ideas or work plans of former colleagues are misappropriated, enormous damage is done not only to the individuals involved but to science in general. A scientist is always given the benefit of the doubt by his colleagues because it can be very difficult to determine whether a particular paper or presentation has violated the code. Science as a field is slow to accuse its members of malfeasance, in large part because scientists don't want to believe that anyone would deliberately destroy either his own reputation or the reputation of science. However, when the evidence is in, scientists are very tough on fraud and abuse of relationships. Those who pursue such dangerous actions are in the end forced from the field.

In the case of the dispute in London over the new class of iron chelators, the outside world saw the young man who appropriated the University College Hospital drug for himself and his new employers as both unwise and impetuous but not dishonest. After all, he had helped to develop the drug in the first place. In fact, the new employers were seen as equally at fault. Outsiders felt that they had rushed prematurely into human trials, exposed patients to unwarranted dangers, and presented results with insufficient care, but this behavior was seen as unpleasant, not an example of misconduct.

As might be expected, the initial results of his clinical trials were encouraging. Then the roof seemed to fall in. A chronically transfused patient with a rare disorder who was well-known both to British and American hematologists tried the drug and became gravely ill. She suddenly lost all of her circulating granulocytes;

these are a class of white cells in the blood responsible for ingesting bacteria. Such a serious complication had never been seen in the decades of experience with Desferal. On the other hand, this untoward reaction is not unknown in therapeutics. There are many approved drugs, particularly those that are used to prevent or treat epilepsy, that are known to cause this complication in a small fraction of the patients who take them. The drug could not be removed from consideration on the basis of this single case. However, the scientific community, distrustful of the investigator and his new hospital, began to say "I told you so."

The next step in the drug's history was even more unfortunate. The young investigator, finding few colleagues in England who wished to work with him, gave the drug, which he had made himself, to a group of physicians in India who used it to treat their patients with thalassemia. This seemed to be the last straw. We were watching an abdication of the responsibility of the investigator for the conduct of clinical investigation. The anger was particularly high in the United States, where the standards for drug evaluation in humans are very rigid. Both the National Institutes of Health and the United States Food and Drug Administration have very clear rules, and several of these rules specifically prevent an investigator from getting around the regulations by dumping an experiment on another country.

An unfortunate example of such dumping occurred in a university hospital in California about fifteen years ago when the recombinant DNA revolution was just beginning. A very bright investigator somehow got the idea that a beta globin gene could be taken up by bone marrow red cells if it was injected directly into the marrow of a thalassemic patient. He further reasoned that the cells would selectively survive if they expressed the gene. This was during the early days of the struggle over the safety of gene research, and the hospital's Human Investigation Committee denied the investigator permission to do the experiment. Their negative opinion was derived in part from their own concerns about its safety and from responses to letters that the committee had sent to other investigators in different institutions. Most replied that the experiment would very likely fail, and they advised against it.

Undaunted, the investigator collaborated with physicians in Italy and in Israel and actually performed the experiments in those countries, where, at the time, annoying Human Investigation Committees did not exist or were not strong enough to stop such activities. The result was a firestorm. When the experiments leaked out, there was a roar of rage from nearly every scientist who had anything to do with molecular biology or thalassemia. The National Institutes of Health promptly moved to take all of its grants away from the investigator; his career in the United States was virtually ruined.

This was a bad loss for American hematology as well as for the investigator. He was then, and remains today, an extremely bright and competent scientist, and he has much to offer the field. He exhibited, however, a serious flaw in judgment. He claimed that he had the interests of dying patients at heart, that the patients had no other option. He thought he would be a hero if the experiments worked. But he failed to comprehend the enormity of flying in the face of the peer review system that researchers must endure if science is to be fairly judged on the basis of quality and if defenseless patients are to be protected from either overzealous or outright unethical physicians. If we are to have a review mechanism that prevents egregious decisions, we must all submit to it or there will be chaos.

The memory of that sad story of the misuse of globin genes by an American physician-scientist in Italy and Israel was much in our minds when we learned that the British investigator of the new orally active chelator had promoted clinical studies in India that would not be permitted in the United States because toxicity studies were incomplete. When stories of serious complications of the drug began to leak from the Indian physicians, most of us thought that the drug was finished. We would have to wait for something better.

Recently one of our former trainees, Nancy Olivieri, now at the Hospital for Sick Children in Toronto, has taken a more positive approach. She was having increasing problems with patients' acceptance of Desferal pumps. Though she was also confident that Desferal, started at an early age and continued at a sensible dose, was both effective and nontoxic, she felt that she had to have an orally active drug, and she needed it now. Nancy and her colleagues decided that the efficacy and toxicity of pyridone had to be determined in a clinical trial, and they persuaded their own excellent chemistry department at the University of Toronto to prepare it very carefully. They then began some cautious trials in Canada, Israel, and Italy. Their initial results are encouraging, though more incidences of granulocyte loss have been observed. More carefully controlled experience will be necessary. It is possible that an orally active drug may be at hand. We will not know for some time, but at least the evaluation is being conducted by responsible and careful doctors who will examine all aspects and report them clearly.

Hope for freedom from the Desferal pump is beginning to rise. I fear, however, that we are still in for some disappointments. An orally active drug may prove more toxic than patients can tolerate, and the frequency of doses required will probably lead to noncompliance by many teenagers and young adults. That has already happened in the Canadian pyridone trial. But we have to persist, we have to be patient, and we have to worry. If we do all three, we will get there.

A New Face

IN MARCH OF 1978, when Dayem was sixteen years old and a somewhat lackadaisical student in a high school in London, he and his mother traveled to Boston to begin treatment with the new device that was all we had to save his life—the subcutaneous Desferal pump.

Dayem looked relatively good to me, though there were plenty of obvious problems. His face, of course, was still very distorted, and he was small for his age and slight of build. Ominously, his skin was deeply bronzed and his liver enlarged. But when I tested his cardiac function by walking rapidly with him up two flights of stairs, his pulse and rate of breathing did not quicken more than mine. After the examination both of us squeezed into a side office in the clinic and began to talk.

"Dayem, I know you hate the Desferal injections, and we both know that they are only partially useful."

"But my mother says you've got a better way to do it."

"Yes, I do, but you may not like it much better. It won't hurt, but you've got to wear a pump every night and have a needle under your skin."

"Where?" he asked.

"Right under the skin of your stomach. The pump with a syringe of Desferal can be mounted in a holster on your belt, and a plastic tube will lead from the syringe under your clothes to the needle. When you go to sleep, the pump can sit on your bedside table."

"You mean I'm tied to the thing all night?"

"That's right."

"What if I want to go dancing or something?"

"Then you can start the pump when you get home, and wear it for the next twelve hours."

He seemed somewhat mollified, but there was something on his mind. He fell silent and looked around the small clinic office without evident curiosity, fixing on nothing in particular. He toyed absently with a stethoscope on the desk. Then he blurted it out. "Doc, I hate the way I look. Everyone stares at me—girls look the other way. Guys do too. I look like a freak. You know it."

His eyes filled with tears. For the first time, the all-encompassing smile was gone. He put his face in his hands and sat hunched up before me, his shoulders shaking. I had never before heard him cry.

If I could have willed him to be handsome, I would have done it then. I wanted to reach out and stroke his ugly face, to hold him to me and tell him that when we both stood up, he would be as fine looking as he wished to be. Instead, I just put my hand on his shoulder and listened to him cry until I could stand it no longer.

"Dayem, you look great to me. When I first met you, I never really thought you could make it to age sixteen. Now here you are. I like your looks and so does everyone who loves you. I'm sorry you don't like your face, but I do. I know who's behind it."

The tears were over. I never saw him cry again. He looked at me with fierce determination. "Yeah doc, I know *you* don't mind how I look, but no one else can stand me outside the family and you. Kids think I'm some sort of freak—I've got to get out of this face, doc. I don't want pity. I want to look decent. You've got to help me."

At that point it dawned on me that he was talking about plastic surgery—that he actually wanted me to arrange a facial reconstruction. Such a bloody and painful operation had been talked about for a few of these misfortunate children, but they didn't live long enough for us to consider it seriously.

"Dayem, to fix your face would mean a huge operation. You'd be in the hospital for weeks. It's an enormous job." I described how the plastic and oral surgeons would have to break the bones in his face and upper jaw and change the shape of his face by taking wedges of bone from both sides of his nose, his cheekbones, and upper jaw, remodeling the structure to set his upper face and jaw in line with his forehead. Then to complete the job in another stage, they would break and extend his lower jaw to match his upper face. It would be a massive and bloody procedure. The recuperation would be very slow. He would be in terrible pain for days after the operation, to say nothing of the risks of infection that were particularly high in him because his spleen had been removed.

He listened intently, nodding occasionally as if to emphasize that he understood every word. It was clear to me that he had made up his mind. I thought of ways that I might reassure him about his appearance, hoping to dissuade him from such a painful and risky ordeal. He seemed to read my mind.

"I don't care. If you want me to live with that stupid pump every night, you've got to do something for me. Fix my face, and then I'll work on the pump."

He looked at me with such deep feeling that I could only take his hand and hold it while we sat there quietly. After a few minutes I asked him to wait for me, and I went out to the waiting room to find his mother.

I brought Mrs. Saif into another clinic room and reported the conversation to her. I hoped that she would oppose such a massive, agonizing, and potentially dangerous undertaking. Instead, she was her usual philosophic self. "We ask so much of him," she pointed out. "He's an adolescent now. He wants to be like other kids. He's not a great student. He is dreaming of being someone, and he can't stand it when people look the other way. He knows they are disgusted and don't want to hurt him. He's tired of being pitied. He needs independence, and it's not going to come from academic work. It's going to come from dealing with people; but he feels like an ugly baby. I know it's a risk. I know it will hurt, but you'll do it here, and he'll be able to face everything else if he feels like a real person, not an ugly reject."

I listened to her carefully. I always do, but I was troubled by a consideration that I did not want to express too bluntly. I had no idea how long Dayem might live. I could not be sure that the new Desferal pump would work for him. Most children with thalassemia are dead or have severe heart disease by age twenty. Why, I thought, should we put him through an excruciating operation only to lose him less than five years later?

As usual, she read my mind. "I know you must be reluctant to put him through something like this when you can't be certain that he will be with us very much longer. But I see the future differently. I want him to be at peace with himself for whatever time he has. I want him to have happiness during those years, and I want him to be self-confident. He needs to feel like someone worth being, if only for a short time."

She was right, of course. Dayem was now a young man with a fierce desire to be like others and, above all, to be independent. I really didn't have any choice. I called Joseph Murray, our chief of plastic surgery.

In 1990 Joe Murray shared the Nobel Prize with Don Thomas for their work on kidney and bone marrow transplantation. Joe was the first surgeon to successfully transplant a kidney, but he is first and foremost a plastic surgeon, committed to the restoration of children with serious malformations. Always considerate and generous with his time, he agreed to meet immediately with Dayem, Mrs. Saif, and me.

"We can do a lot to improve your appearance, Dayem," he said with his Yankee firmness. "But it will be tough in the post-operative period." Joe looked hard at Dayem. "You understand that it will be difficult for you in the first few weeks after the procedure. It's going to be painful and slow-going for a while."

Dayem gazed carefully at him, and then said softly, "I want my face changed, Dr. Murray." The die was cast. Dayem would have a new face.

Before the procedure, I wanted to be sure of Dayem's response to subcutaneous Desferal. If he was to take the risk of facial surgery, I wanted to be more confident that the new treatment would reduce his immediate likelihood of death from iron overload. To my disappointment, Dayem was not one of our best responders. He certainly excreted much more iron after the subcutaneous dose than after an intramuscular dose, but compared with others, his rate of excretion remained modest on a standard dose. I would need to increase it if he was to have a daily iron excretion that would place him in a substantial negative iron balance. To do so, I adjusted his daily dose until we found one that would remove the iron that we continued to give him in transfusions, and, as well, remove some iron from the large pool that had collected in him before the subcutaneous chelation with Desferal had begun.

I found the correct dose with little effort, but Dayem began to complain of pain, redness, and itching at the subcutaneous site. That was another disappointment. Sensitivity to Desferal had occurred in one or two of our patients, but it had been easily overcome by the addition of small doses of a corticosteroid-like drug to the Desferal. In Dayem's case the addition of the steroid made a difference, but it was not entirely successful. He still complained about discomfort, though he said it was tolerable. He returned to Europe to get used to the new method of Desferal treatment after he and his mother had made arrangements to come back in three months for the facial surgery.

In July of 1978 Dayem and his mother returned. I had one more long talk with Dayem to be certain that he fully understood the seriousness of his decision. He was, if anything, more determined than ever, so I acted as optimistic as I could, shook his hand, and told him that I would see him on the morning of the operation. I asked one of our best trainees to keep a special eye on Dayem and be sure that nothing was overlooked during the post-operative period. Then I waited.

The surgery began in the late morning. It was carried out by Murray and the oral surgeons with whom he had worked in similar kinds of cases, if not in this particular disease. Together, they had made careful measurements of Dayem's face and had created a mold of what they wished to achieve. With the model before them, they began the bloody process of cracking the bones in his face, nose, and upper jaw, remodeling his nose, and pushing the loose parts backward until the ugly protuberances were less apparent. Blood gushed from the fractured nose and the cracked cheekbones. The hugely expanded bone marrow spaces bled copiously. The anesthesiologists had to pour blood into him to sustain his blood pressure. All of our careful calculations about his transfusion schedule during the operation were ignored as the surgical team struggled to keep him alive while they fixed his face. As Murray deftly repaired the fractures, the oral surgeons wired Dayem's upper jaw together and checked to be sure that his airway was open. Six hours later, his face swathed in bandages, he returned to the recovery area to begin a slow convalescence.

The pain must have been dreadful. He required reasonably heavy doses of narcotics, but he would not complain. In fact, he seemed happier every day.

To my amazement he absolutely sailed through the post-op period, though he had plenty of pain and general discomfort. The worst complication was a collection of blood at the sites of the fractures, particularly those of the upper jaw. As the blood slowly decayed, his mouth smelled so bad that he became nauseated; however, true to his name, he surmounted all the problems and was discharged in less than two weeks. I remembered then the resident who stated on Dayem's first admission that the boy must have nine lives. Dayem had made all my fears seem groundless.

There is something about determination in a patient that changes the results of a procedure. Every doctor who has to use a difficult treatment or manage very ill patients has seen the effects of a patient's attitude and confidence on the outcome. We don't understand mind-body connections very well because they are so difficult to study with acceptably quantitative methods. We know, however, that confidence and will often seem to make an enormous difference. Joe Murray's approach to Dayem was one of calm confidence in the procedure itself and in its benefit to this particular young man. Dayem wanted the procedure desperately and threw in his lot with Murray. I believe, though I will never be able to prove it, that the relationship between the two of them, and the support provided by the surgical nurses who had taken many patients through such procedures, made a huge clinical difference. Dayem left Boston with his jaw and cheekbones wired together, but he would soon have the new face he so badly wanted.

Six weeks later, he returned for removal of the wires and some orthodontic procedures that would restore his bite. His face was still too swollen and black and blue to know how he would look, but he insisted that he saw improvement already. Again, his determination was very evident. A few months later, pictures began to arrive that confirmed every one of Dayem's beliefs. He was achieving a normal appearance.

He looked marvelous at his next check-up. In fact he had become absolutely handsome by anyone's standards. Joe Murray made some critical measurements of the angles formed by Dayem's forehead, nose, and chin and decided that the lower jaw lengthening would not be necessary. He would look good without that nasty additional operation. I was delighted and so was Dayem and his family. The days when girls looked the other way were coming to an end, but my most serious difficulties with him were just beginning.

The fact that teenagers do not cooperate well with complex or chronic medical regimes is almost a cliché in the medical world. But Dayem had an additional issue. Not only did he hate the Desferal treatment because it was inconvenient, embarrassing, and interfered with his nightlife; he also found it uncomfortable. The redness and pain at every injection site continued; or so he claimed. Furthermore, he had one episode of serious infection; nearly half an ounce of pus was drained from one infected site. His abdominal skin looked normal, but I had to admit that after each nightly injection, there was more redness and hardness at the site than we saw in most patients. I reassured him and sent him back to Europe to continue the subcutaneous Desferal, but he hated the method and feared another infection. He said that he didn't mind wearing the pump. In fact, he enjoyed showing it off to his friends. "It's cool," they would say, but the skin irritation and the need to wear it every night bothered him tremendously.

In 1979 Mr. Saif moved with his family from London to Arlington, Virginia, a suburb of Washington. He became the chief executive officer of the United States branch of his company for the next four years. Dayem had finished high school in London and started university classes in Washington, attending for only two or three weeks before dropping out for good. He wanted to be independent more than he wanted to read books, but he simply hadn't figured out what he would do with himself.

As far as my medical care plans were concerned, I thought they were very well organized. He would receive his blood transfusions at the National Institutes of Health, and the excellent hematology program in the National Heart, Lung and Blood Institute at NIH would provide emergency care if needed. He would come to Boston regularly for evaluations and adjustments as necessary. How critical the back-up of the NHLBI hematologists was to Dayem's survival became clear when he contracted severe viral meningitis and encephalitis. The excellent care he received from my colleagues there allowed him to recover without any neurologic defects.

Though I initially believed that Dayem's proximity would make my treatment more effective, those were to be four difficult and sometimes contentious years in my relationship with him.

DAYEM THREW DOWN the gauntlet during his evaluation in Boston in July of 1979. He was then seventeen years old and interested in (in descending order) girls, making money, popular music, cars, and any electronic device other than his Desferal pump. One day he arrived at Children's for a detailed inpatient evaluation looking like a bronzed matinee idol surrounded by a gang of teenagers who were dressed in the latest fashions and who spread themselves liberally all over his bed. At night they would shut the door and draw the curtains. None of us knew exactly what was going on in that room, but it sounded like a bacchanal. After each party Dayem would sleep until noon. His indolent life angered me, particularly when he stated unequivocally that he hated the pump and the subcutaneous injections, that he hadn't in fact touched the pump in two months, and that he had given himself an occasional intramuscular injection but wanted nothing more to do with the whole chelation business.

I was livid. I wanted to shake him. Whatever skills I may have acquired from dealing with my own children seemed to abandon me. Dayem was doing to me what a physician can never allow: he was getting me good and mad. Indeed, I could practically taste my own self-pity. I had helped to develop a very useful treatment program with this young man very much in mind, a program that was being hailed as a major advance around the world, and he was coolly telling me that he wasn't interested. Nubile teenaged girls lay all over his hospital bed while Dayem challenged every rule we had and thought up brilliant ways to defy me.

"Who's in charge here?" I moaned to myself. "These kids are taking over, and this guy is basically telling me to take my treatment program and stuff it. Am I supposed to stand here and just accept this?"

Cleverly, I believe, Mrs. Saif didn't come along on this particular trip. In fact, she began making it a policy to stay away, telling me that it was my relationship with him that mattered now. She could no longer be an effective manager of my plans because Dayem was giving her as hard a time as he was giving me.

For a year, it was a standoff. Dayem would use the pump rarely and only when I called and virtually screamed at him over the phone. He stopped the intramuscular injections because, as he would mischievously point out, "You say they're no good anyway, doc."

"They're not good *enough*," I would nearly roar, "but they're better than nothing."

Something about his insouciance really got to me. The fact is that he had cheated me. "Look Dayem, when I agreed to that big facial surgery, we made a deal. You would get a new face, and I was supposed to get your cooperation. Well, Joe Murray did his thing, your face is terrific, and all I'm getting is a constant battle with you over the most basic things. You're eighteen, and you won't see twenty-one if you don't cooperate the way you said you would."

It was a mawkish and ridiculous scene. Here was this teenager who had been chronically ill for the first seven years of life happening upon sexual adventure and a bit of independence for the first time; and here was this New England born and bred pediatrician, who saw himself as a major contributor to a field and was accustomed to being promptly heeded, drawing himself up huffily and demanding the sanctity of prior agreements. I would have laughed hard had I been watching through the window, but I was part of it, and I was extremely upset and disappointed. Short of imprisoning him and tying him down, there was no way I could achieve what I wanted. Finally, seeing that anger and hurt were going to get me nowhere, I tried a friendly, therapeutic approach. I decided to be understanding of Dayem's new-found adolescent life and to see whether he would be willing to explore the issue of why he continued to refuse treatment even though he admitted that failure to take the treatment would kill him. I referred him for counseling to an excellent psychologist in Washington, but he discontinued his meetings with the therapist after a handful of sessions.

Soon after, I wrote him a pompous, appeasing, almost treacly-sounding letter. "Your lack of compliance with Desferal," I wrote, "is worrisome, though understandable. As you are aware, it is often very hard to impose restrictions on young people, especially when they have great intellectual capacity and a tremendous desire to enjoy life and to live." Then I couldn't resist a dig. "Love doth make fools of us all," I quoted. Finally, I pointed out that there was a small and possibly inconsequential change in his electrocardiogram. I suggested that the test should be repeated. I hoped that the news would sufficiently alarm him. It didn't.

In 1981 when Dayem was nearly nineteen, I knew I was in for a tremendous and nearly continuous battle with him. He was getting into every adolescent scourge that I could name and, I was certain, a few I didn't know much about. Marijuana looked tame. There was enough cocaine around Washington to refer to the place as the "District of Colombia." I would regularly accuse Dayem and his buddies of being the chief customers and tradespeople of the Medellín cartel. He would deny any such thing. "A few experiments, Doc. What do you want? Don't you do experiments?"

What Dayem did admit to was an overwhelming desire to be his own man. He was into almost any activity that would give him financial independence. He was alternately a car salesman (including bulletproof limousines), a clothing salesman, or a salesman of practically anything else. Then there were the young ladies. I stopped counting them after a while. There were also car accidents. Indeed, the fracture period temporarily recurred when he broke his ankle in one wreck. Nothing was wrong with his bones, but plenty was wrong with his driving and that of his companions.

Despite the fact that Dayem was doing nothing we told him to do except taking his transfusions, careful cardiac examinations did not reveal any serious abnormalities. But I was very concerned that his failure to accept the Desferal treatment would inevitably lead to heart disease. Therefore, I decided to re-admit him to the Clinical Research Center at Children's and have another serious conversation with him about his options.

"Dayem," I began, "if you don't take the subcutaneous Desferal, you'll get heart disease and die. You know that, don't you?"

He nodded slowly.

"So if you refuse, we've got to do something else. There are only two options. We can search for a related or even an unrelated matched donor for a bone marrow transplant. Now, you know how dangerous a marrow transplant can be. In the best of circumstances right now, at least 20 percent of patients die in the first year. That's with a matched sibling donor, and your siblings don't match. In your case, the risk is at least a 40 percent chance of dying in the first year after a transplant from a matched unrelated donor. Furthermore, we've yet to transplant a thalassemic patient here, because so far all our patients have preferred the pump to the risk of a transplant. A safer approach would be your second option: to put a semipermanent catheter in one of your veins and pump in Desferal continuously. It would be the same kind of a catheter that we make for patients who have to be on regular dialysis for kidney disease. That at least will stop the discomfort from injections."

He looked at me very seriously. I knew I was getting somewhere with him, but I couldn't keep the frustration out of my voice. "You've got to make a choice. And let me tell you, my friend, you're not going to die on *my* watch. When I first met you, I told your family that we were going to find a way to give you a decent life. I'm going to keep that promise, and neither you nor anybody else is going to stop me." Suddenly I was raising my voice. "You'll sit in this damned hospital room until you make up your mind about what you want—a marrow transplant, or intravenous Desferal that you'll receive through a catheter. So pick your approach. It's your decision, but *you're going to make a decision.* We're not sitting around any longer while you slowly kill yourself. And by the way, in case you want some help with the transplant decision, go down the hall and look at the kid in the last room on the right."

That last flourish, I admit, was unfair to everyone. The poor teenager in that room had had a marrow transplant for leukemia from an unrelated donor and had developed terrible graft-versus-host disease. His skin was ravaged, he was severely jaundiced, and he had nearly intractable diarrhea. He was slowly and miserably dying.

Dayem spent that early evening standing outside the windows that separate the sterile transplant rooms from the corridor of the ward. He talked to the nurses who were caring for the transplanted young boy. The next day Dayem asked to see me. He had devoted much of the night from midnight to four in the morning talking to one of the nurses who knew him very well. He had made a decision to take the drug by pump if it was given by the intravenous catheter rather than a subcutaneous injection.

I told him that he had made a wise choice. Though the intravenous catheter approach would not be easy and was certainly not free of serious problems, including infection and clotting, unrelated matched transplants were still very risky. I insisted that he commit himself to a very long stay in the hospital, where we could use an ordinary intravenous infusion to find an optimal dose of Desferal that would clean out a substantial part of the iron he had accumulated during his long period of noncompliance. In that way, we might make some real headway against heart disease.

Dayem agreed. He stayed with us in the Clinical Research Center for a month, and for that entire time we infused him with intravenous Desferal around the clock. He eliminated grams of iron. Even Dayem seemed pleased with his deep red urine. Furthermore, he noticed that his skin began to lighten, and he was feeling less fatigued. We were making progress in dealing with that toxic pool of free iron.

Toward the end of the stay, we had another conversation. "Look, doc," he said, "I've been stupid; give me another chance with the injections. I'll give it a real try. I've talked some more about the catheter idea and I'm scared it will get infected or clot. Honestly, I'll take the stupid needle seriously."

I was truly delighted. "You're on, my friend. Let's get you out of here. Go back to Washington, make money, start the Desferal, and let's see where we stand. If it isn't tolerable, we'll give you an IV catheter."

We shook hands on it. I had made a new deal with Dayem, or so I hoped. But in my heart I was beginning to lose faith in Desferal for him. I knew he had regularly fobbed me off with promises. If I was to help this young man, and many like him, I would have to be successful in the second and much slower-moving prong of my pincer attack—the development of a molecular treatment that could be as effective as a successful marrow transplant without the risk of graft-versus-host disease. This would require a massive basic investigation into hemoglobin gene behavior. Our laboratory and others had already set about to attack that task.

Banned in Boston

WHEN DAYEM LEFT the Clinical Research Center at Children's on that day in 1981, I walked slowly through the hospital on my way to the hematology research laboratory. I realized that we could develop a truly effective treatment for Dayem, and patients like him, only by understanding the molecular basis of the genetic problem, and at that moment we were already well on the way to its solution.

My first approach to thalassemia at the molecular level had begun in the late 1960s, when my colleagues and I measured the relative rates at which alpha, beta, and gamma globin chains are produced (synthesized) in red cells. The techniques we used were modifications of those described by John Clegg and David Weatherall in the early 1960s. What we learned was that alpha and beta chains are produced at very nearly equal rates in the red cells of normal individuals, and there is little or no synthesis of gamma chains. In most patients with severe thalassemia, however, we found little or no production of beta chains, variable rates of gamma chain production, and normal alpha chain production, all of which adds up to a severe imbalance in the formation of globin chains. However, in a few patients with milder forms of thalassemia, we detected unusually high levels of gamma chain production. This permitted these patients to make large amounts of fetal hemoglobin which could fill their red blood cells and help the cells survive the attack of rubbish-eating cells in the marrow, spleen, and liver. We made every effort to understand how these rare patients could make so much fetal hemoglobin. If we could unlock their secret, we might be able to activate that capacity in other patients, through gene transfer or drug therapy.

Hoping to find some mitigating feature of Dayem's case such as an increased capacity to produce gamma chains, we had measured the rate of globin chain synthesis in the developing red cells in his blood and bone marrow and in the cells of his parents. Unfortunately, we detected nothing unusual. The only encouraging finding was the fact that Dayem's cells could produce a small amount of normal beta chain. One or both of his defective beta genes could actually function, albeit at a low level. By that time, we were classifying the beta thalassemia genes as either beta zero or beta plus. The beta zero genes were incapable of any beta globin production, while the beta plus genes evinced a detectable if low level of beta chain production. Dayem was classified as a beta plus, although the absolute amount of beta chain that he could accumulate in his red cells was extremely small. Furthermore, he was not a very substantial producer of gamma chains. Most of the hemoglobin in his blood was fetal hemoglobin, but the total amount that he could effectively produce was very low. That was why he came to us originally with only a little more than one gram of hemoglobin in each 100 milliliters of his blood. As far as we could tell in the early 1970s, when we made that measurement on Dayem and his family, he was an uncomplicated severe beta plus thalassemic.

We would need the techniques of molecular genetics, including recombinant DNA technology, to explain his genetic defects more completely, and those were not to become available until the following decade. That was why we had devoted most of our attention to the complexities of his treatment program, including removal of his spleen, transfusion, and iron chelation with Desferal.

As we considered how we might best use our laboratory resources to advance our basic understanding of thalassemia and, in Dayem's case, determine the precise defect in his beta globin genes, Bernie Forget (a young trainee who was on duty for consultations in hematology during a particularly busy week in 1970) walked into the laboratory with a blood smear of a newborn infant in his hand.

Forget told me that the baby, Maureen, was very anemic, and most of her few circulating red cells contained nuclei. That sounded a lot like Rh disease, but Bernie had already shown that the baby had no anti-Rh antibodies, and her blood group was compatible with that of her mother. We had to consider other causes.

Together, we took a careful look at Maureen's blood smear through the microscope. The red cells were relatively few in number, and many were nucleated, but I noticed something else. They contained far less hemoglobin than normal. Since Maureen had never bled, this seemed to be a case of thalassemia that had begun during fetal life. Obviously it couldn't be beta thalassemia because that disease does not become apparent until the infant is about six months old, when the beta globin genes that are supposed to switch on fail to do so.

In newborns, the gamma chains produced before the "beta switch" pair up with the alpha chains to make fetal hemoglobin. Perhaps Maureen has a form of *alpha* thalassemia, we thought. But she was of English and Scottish stock, and severe alpha thalassemia in fetuses and newborns had been observed thus far solely in Asians. To be certain, Forget, Kan, and I examined her hemoglobin very closely and found no evidence of that disease. This was not alpha thalassemia.

It wasn't beta thalassemia, and it wasn't alpha thalassemia. Could this be a form of *gamma* thalassemia? Such a condition had never been previously reported. We knew that there were two gamma genes upstream of the single delta and beta genes on each chromosome 11. Could Maureen have lost the function of two or more of them? To make that measurement, we would have to measure globin chain synthesis in the baby's blood and in the blood of her parents. But before embarking on that task, we examined her parents' red cells. Sure enough, her father's blood was not normal. He had small red cells with less than a normal amount of hemoglobin in them, and he remembered that his parents had told him that he had been so anemic at birth that he had required a transfusion! We were clearly onto something new, a type of thalassemia that had never been previously described, and one which might have enormous implications for treating many other types of thalassemia.

Kan and I immediately measured the rates of synthesis of Maureen's globin chains and found that her gamma chain production was considerably lower than we expected for a two-day-old baby. Her beta chain production—and even her delta chain production—was very much lower than expected as well. But in fact our expectations were just educated guesses; we didn't really know much about rates of synthesis in newborns. We needed a comparative measurement from a healthy newborn baby of the same age—that is, we needed a control. Where would we get it? We couldn't use the blood of our babies in the hospital nursery: they were there because they were sick. We couldn't put painful needles in the veins of newborns in the well-baby nursery at the new Brigham and Women's Hospital across the street: that would be unethical.

Slowly, Forget and I fixed our eyes on Kan. His wife, Alvera (my former lab technician), had given birth to their second daughter just three days before. The perfect control was literally in Kan's hands. We had only to persuade Alvera to let him take a blood sample from baby Debbie and all would be well.

But who should ask Alvera? She is a marvelous, generous person, but more than once I had encountered her Latin temperament during our years together in the lab. The safest strategy, I thought, was to let Kan pop the question. If she threw him out of the house, we would know that the answer was negative.

The next morning Kan came into the lab clutching a small tube of Debbie's blood. After minimal fireworks, Alvera had reluctantly agreed, mainly because she trusted his technique. He does have good hands.

The results of the comparison were very impressive. Maureen and her father had definite evidence of beta chain deficiency, and even her gamma chain production was much lower than Debbie Kan's. We proposed that Maureen must have inherited a large deletion of the globin genes on one of her chromosome 11's from her father. Both gamma genes, the delta gene, and the beta gene, we suggested, must be missing on that chromosome. Maureen's hemoglobin production depended on the output of the genes on the other, unaffected, chromosome. But they could not keep up with the increased demands for hemoglobin that the fetus, in its relatively oxygen-starved state, makes on the marrow. The only possible response of Maureen's marrow to her reduced oxygen-carrying capacity was to produce red cells at a maximal rate. Out they came into the blood, still carrying nuclei in their rush to provide relief. As Maureen matured and the switch from gamma genes to beta genes was completed, she no longer required gamma chains, and her red cells became no different than those of her father, whose blood looked exactly like that of other people with ordinary beta thalassemia trait.

A decade later, I revisited this case with Stuart Orkin, who had joined our laboratory as a trainee at the beginning of the molecular biology revolution and remains with us as the Leland Fikes Professor of Pediatrics and an investigator of the Howard Hughes Medical Institute. A member of the National Academy of Sciences, he is now one of the most distinguished experimental hematologists in the world. Using recombinant DNA techniques, Stuart analyzed Maureen's DNA and that of her father and confirmed that there was indeed a very large deletion of all of the globin genes on one copy of chromosome 11. Several other cases with similar deletions were soon reported from around the world. The disease is now called gamma-delta-beta thalassemia.

As Forget, Kan, and I were readying the first case of gamma-delta-beta thalassemia for publication, we realized that some of our conclusions, though exciting and novel, were more inferential than truly solid. After all, our only control was the blood of Debbie Kan. Debbie is certainly a normal, healthy young woman today, but her rates of beta and gamma globin chain synthesis in the neonatal period might not have been representative of every baby. There might be, we correctly reasoned, a rather wide distribution among normal babies if enough of them could be studied.

Furthermore, an exciting idea had grasped Kan and me which would require a much broader data base. If we were correct in our diagnosis of baby Maureen's condition on the first day of her life, why not try to diagnose thalassemia in fetuses within the first or second trimester of gestation? If we could develop a safe and accurate way to provide prenatal diagnosis to women at risk for thalassemia, perhaps we could contribute to a reduction of the caseload in the Mediterranean communities in which the disease was so common. Of course we realized that many of the families at risk were either Roman Catholic or Greek Orthodox and might not even consider prenatal diagnosis, much less selective abortion, but we decided to determine first whether there was any useful technical approach to the problem before we concerned ourselves with religious or political aspects of fetal research.

Our initial task was to collect several samples of umbilical cord blood from normal newborns and measure globin chain synthesis in their red cells. This gave us a valuable index of the expected ratios of beta and gamma chain production at birth. To measure the progress of the switch from gamma to beta genes, we also needed to establish a ratio of beta chain to gamma chain synthesis in fetuses of different gestational ages. As the fetus ages and approaches the time of birth, we reasoned, the beta to gamma ratio should progressively, and then sharply, increase. But to confirm our hunch, we needed blood samples from properly timed fetuses.

Kan and I discussed the matter with members of the Obstetrics Department at Boston City Hospital. Physicians there were performing second-trimester abortions by instilling a hormone called prostaglandin into the pregnant woman's intrauterine cavity. The hormone induces premature labor, from which the very young fetus does not survive. Our first task was to collect a few samples of cord blood from prostaglandin-induced abortions.

Dr. Kenneth Edelin, the first black chief resident in obstetrics in the history of Boston City Hospital, usually performed these second-trimester abortions, and through him we were able to obtain our precious cell samples. In the laboratory at Children's, we added a small amount of an amino acid carrying a radioactive tracer to incubate with the cells before we separated the globin chains, and then we began to analyze them. To our delight, there was always a small but clearly detectable fraction of radioactive beta chain and easily detectable gamma and alpha chain radioactivity. Since the uptake of radioactive amino acid told us that new chains were being synthesized, we now knew that a small but detectable amount of beta globin is made in the second trimester of human fetal development.

One of the blood samples we received was from a first-trimester fetus. Its estimated gestational age was ten weeks. In that sample, there were two radioactive peaks in beta chain production. One was clearly from normal beta chain production, but the second was from sickle beta chain production. This fetus, we knew, was the product of a union of two black parents. Clearly, one of them had sickle cell trait and had passed it to this fetus. We had detected sickle trait in a ten-week fetus! If we could do that, we hoped that it would also be possible to detect thalassemia in a first-trimester fetus by finding that the peak of normal beta chain radioactivity was much lower than normal. The technical problem facing us was daunting, however. The normal ratio of beta to gamma globin chain synthesis is a little less than 10 percent in a first-trimester fetus. How could we reliably detect a further reduction? To do so, we would have to determine the range of normal values in a substantial number of fetuses of various developmental ages. Even if we could securely distinguish severe thalassemia from normal in a fetus, our challenge was to provide measurements accurate enough to distinguish severe thalassemic fetuses from fetuses with mere thalassemia trait. The latter is an innocuous diagnosis and certainly, in and of itself, not an indication for abortion.

At this point two events diverted my attention. First, Kan decided to accept a fine research position at the University of California in San Francisco. It was hard to say goodbye to him and Alvera, because I had worked closely with them for years and knew I would miss them terribly. But the move was very good for both of them. An important part of my job is to train research hematologists for academic medical centers around the world. In doing so, I train my own competition. Kan was one of the very best young faculty members in my experience, and I realized that I could not hold on to him forever. Indeed, Kan went on to an extraordinary career that brought him to the very top of medical genetics in this country and around the world.

The second distraction was far more serious and was to occupy much of my attention in the following months. The *Roe v. Wade* decision by the United States Supreme Court had severely reduced the capacity of the states to limit a woman's choice to have an abortion. The response of those who opposed the decision was predictable. Various groups, some sponsored by the Roman Catholic Church or other religious persuasions, some highly conservative and others anti-establishment, were galvanized into action to overturn *Roe v. Wade,* to harass women seeking abortions, or to attack clinics that provided this service. The obstetric unit at Boston City Hospital was a major target for them.

THE BATTLE BEGAN when the district attorney of Suffolk County, where Boston City is located, carried out a raid on the hospital's Pathology Department. Guided by a disgruntled hospital employee, he found the remains of fetuses in preservative jars. Witnesses came forward to state that Dr. Edelin had murdered the fetuses—that they had been born alive and he had not supported them but rather had actively contributed to their death. Here was the perfect setup: one or two white nurses pitted against a black physician. It was a politician's nightmare and a rabble rouser's delight. The right-to-lifers were not stupid, however. They knew they could count on the district attorney to get an indictment against Edelin, because in Boston there was more than enough anti-black feeling to persuade a grand jury that a crime might have been committed. But a conviction was another matter. The evidence against Edelin was ridiculous. Medical testimony would be solidly behind him. A rational judge would throw the case out of court.

Enter Mildred Jefferson, M.D., the daughter of a military chaplain, the first black woman graduate of Harvard Medical School, and a trained surgeon to boot. Attractive, intelligent, and above all a remarkably effective public speaker, Jefferson came to the trial to testify against Edelin. Though the scientific testimony of a score of witnesses was all in favor of Edelin, he was convicted of manslaughter.

Not long thereafter, Edelin's conviction was overturned on appeal. That was a better day, though the struggle about abortion and research on fetuses was to become unbearable in Massachusetts.

The site of the next major conflict about abortion and medical research was, again, Boston City Hospital. Infectious disease specialists there were faced with increasing numbers of pregnant patients with life-threatening intrauterine infections that required high doses of antibiotics. Yet there was little or no information about the passage of antibiotics across the placenta into the fetus, much less any data about which specific antibiotics might be the most or the least effective.

To gain reliable data on these questions, physicians (with appropriate consent) gave women who were about to have elective abortions a dose of a particular antibiotic, and then later they measured the antibiotic levels in the aborted fetus. The article describing their findings was published in the *New England Journal of Medicine,* and when it became public, right-to-life groups went into a frenzy. They demanded a criminal investigation, but there was no law on the books that could possibly make the doctors' actions a crime. Having no law with which to prosecute, the right-to-lifers decided to create one. With the help of a Boston College Law School professor, they crafted a draconian fetal research law that would prevent the use of fetal tissue for any kind of research at all. The bill was introduced into the state legislature by an otherwise liberal young representative who was well liked by his colleagues. It seemed certain of passage.

While all of this was going on in the legislature, I was paying no attention to fetal research laws or any other political issues. I was working instead with my young associates on the problem of detecting thalassemia in the first trimester and at the very least within the first twenty weeks of pregnancy. I needed to analyze the aborted fetuses of women with thalassemia trait whose partners were men with thalassemia trait. Those fetuses would have a one-in-four chance of having severe thalassemia, a one-in-two chance of having thalassemia trait, and a one-in-four chance of being entirely normal. To acquire the appropriate samples, I needed to find a clinic that saw a large number of women with thalassemia trait, because many of these women, I knew, abort every pregnancy out of fear that they might have a child with this dreadful disease.

I found the right source in London at the University College Hospital, where Ernst Huehns and Bernadette Modell were respectively in charge of the hematology laboratory and the thalassemia clinic. Huehns had been interested for some time in the development of hemoglobin in human fetuses and had already developed some methods which had revealed that beta chain synthesis might be detectable in the first trimester. Modell was then, and remains, a remarkably devoted clinician who was one of the first to organize the care of the increasing flood of thalassemic patients who were then entering England, largely as a result of the civil war in Cyprus. She was also one of the first European clinicians to recognize the importance of maintaining a high level of hemoglobin in thalassemic patients through appropriate transfusion techniques. When our method of subcutaneous Desferal therapy was described, she was among the first to apply it in patients in the U.K.

The three of us struck up an excellent collaboration, and soon first-trimester blood samples were traveling across the Atlantic. Nothing about this was illegal, but it was a bit difficult to explain what the samples were to the customs agents in Boston's Logan Airport. Neither "fetus" nor "blood" was a particularly acceptable term to that suspicious breed. But my technicians and research fellows do not look like drug kingpins, vampires, or illicit abortionists, and the packages bearing their precious vials, marked with the innocuous label "medical sample," made their way to the lab.

The first blood sample we tested was from an eight-week fetus. There were only two or three drops of blood. We made our measurement and found that there *was* a radioactive beta chain peak that was about 7 percent of the gamma chain peak. We looked that up on a graph that I had prepared with Gabriel Cividalli (now chief of Pediatric Hematology at Hadassah Hospital in Jerusalem). It showed the beta-to-gamma ratios from our fetal blood study conducted with obstetricians at Boston City Hospital. The value in the eight-week fetus appeared to be normal. The next two samples were also normal. Both fetuses were aborted by women with thalassemia trait who were married to a normal man. Since there was a 50 percent chance that the fetus would be normal, we still did not know whether our methods would detect thalassemia in the fetus even if it was present.

The next two samples were more exciting. In these, women with thalassemia trait were married to men with the same diagnosis. Here was the genetic condition we needed. In these matings, there was a 50 percent chance that the fetus would have beta thalassemia trait and a 25 percent chance that the fetus would either have severe beta thalassemia or be entirely normal. The first sample was from a ten-week fetus. The radioactivity in the beta chains was only 4 percent of the radioactivity in the gamma chains. This was certainly indicative of beta thalassemia trait. But the next sample was what we were waiting for. There was no radioactivity at all in the beta chains. The only radioactivity was in the gamma and the alpha chains. This fetus surely had severe beta thalassemia. The case strongly supported our idea that severe beta thalassemia could be detected in the first trimester and could even be discriminated from beta thalassemia trait.

We were very excited by these findings, but we remained cautious. The data, though very supportive, didn't prove that our method would really work in practice. That would require a clinical trial. We would have to see whether we could actually make these diagnoses in living fetuses. If our methods were truly reliable, we should find severe disease in 25 percent of fetuses resulting from matings between two people with thalassemia trait. Furthermore, follow-up studies in newborns who were *not* aborted should confirm our prenatal diagnoses. Only by such a large analysis in an actual trial could the method prove itself. Now we had the preliminary data that would allow us to proceed with such a trial.

A major stumbling block was yet to be faced, however. All of these prenatal measurements required a sample of the fetus's red cells, but a safe and reliable method for acquiring fetal blood during pregnancy had not yet been developed. Furthermore, any sample of fetal blood was likely to be contaminated with maternal blood. Those maternal cells would produce beta chains because the mothers had thalassemia trait, not severe disease. If there were enough maternal cells present in the sample, the beta chain production in those cells might lead to a false diagnosis of beta thalassemia trait in a fetus which in fact had severe disease.

Prenatal diagnosis has always been dogged by the risks of false negatives and false positives. In the false negative error described above, the pregnancy of a fetus with a serious illness is not interrupted because the mother is persuaded by the test that the fetus is healthy. The mother, who has relied on her physicians to spare her and her family the agony of caring for a chronically ill child, is then crushed with an unwanted responsibility that she had tried in the most serious way to avoid.

A false positive diagnosis is perhaps a greater burden on the physician. The entire concept of prenatal diagnosis and *selective* abortion is to avoid abortion in the majority of pregnancies and to carry out the unpleasant procedure only when it is medically indicated. Women with thalassemia trait married to men with thalassemia trait often interrupt *all* pregnancies, particularly after they have given birth to a child with severe disease. They just cannot afford to take the 25 percent chance that lightning will strike again in their lives (see figure 7 on page 57). Many are eager for prenatal diagnosis if the procedure can nearly guarantee them a healthy fetus. They are likely to abort if there is any doubt. A false positive diagnosis is therefore very apt to lead to the abortion of a healthy fetus—an unhappy result after a great deal of effort, and a breakdown of the compact between the physician and the patient.

This dilemma is a classical example of the influence of technology on medical ethics. The most important way to achieve high ethical standards in medicine is to employ excellent technology that is reliable and predictable. Though certain ethicists might disagree, I believe that many ethical decisions in medicine depend on the quality of the technology available. As technology improves, the application of ethical standards has to change with it. It is unethical to raise the hopes of a pregnant woman and offer a diagnostic method that is unreliable. It is very ethical to do one's best to help such a woman with a painful decision if, and only if, the techniques that one offers are reliable and safe.

I discussed that issue carefully with Mrs. Saif on several occasions because I had come to rely on her judgment and sense of fairness. In her opinion, a physician's ethical code must satisfy the individual needs of patients. A code that would deny information to a woman who wants to know the state of health of her fetus could not be ethical in any sense. If the woman chooses to interrupt her pregnancy after she has gained that information, neither the physician nor anyone else should try to impede her. She was very certain that the decision must be personal and not societal.

Whether Mrs. Saif herself would ever contemplate an abortion was unclear in her mind. Many years later, she had this to say about the ethical dilemma she would face if she had to make a decision about selective abortion: "Let's imagine that today I am pregnant, and I have a prenatal diagnosis. I want this child, but they tell me this fetus has thalassemia major. Thirty years ago I would have chosen abortion at once. Today the dilemma would be huge because I know how wonderful Dayem is, how much he means to me and others. Am I allowed to give birth to a child who is going to suffer, just because I now know how much that child can be enriching to others and himself? That's the dilemma I would have to face. I would have to decide between the suffering of the child and how much the child can bring to others. Most probably I would ask Dayem what to do. I would ask him whether life is worth living at whatever the cost. Thank God that I cannot have children anymore. I wouldn't want to make that decision."

During the months that we were developing prenatal diagnostic techniques, I also asked Mrs. Saif whether my focus on the prevention of thalassemia was repugnant to her. Did she believe that my efforts should instead be directed toward the treatment of the living? Her response was typical of her. "You should do today what it is possible to do. You don't know how to cure this disease. You will someday, we hope, but you can't do it now. You should do the best you can for Dayem, other patients, and other families. If one of the contributions you can make is to prevent new cases, you should work hard on that. Those who are living with the disease now should certainly understand and applaud." A few months later, when I found myself in bitter public debates about fetal research, I remembered what she said and gained strength from her support.

WHILE the contentious ethical issues surrounding fetal research were being debated, my laboratory focused on two technical problems. We had to find a way to acquire a small sample of fetal blood without injury to the fetus, and, if there were maternal cells in the sample, we had to get rid of them. The latter proved to be relatively simple. Colleagues at Johns Hopkins had shown that fetal cells are resistant to swelling and rupturing in certain salt solutions that cause adult cells to burst. Using this technique, Dr. Blanche Alter—then a young trainee and now chief of pediatric hematology at the University of Texas at Galveston—and I could then capture the unbroken cells and be confident that they were from the fetus and not the mother.

The biggest problem facing us was the acquisition of a good sample of fetal blood without injury to the fetus or to the mother. For that purpose, obstetricians needed to develop a method that they had never used before. The instrument of choice is called a fetoscope. It is a tiny telescope with a light source and a needle attached to it. The scope can be inserted under ultrasound guidance into the pregnant uterus, and a vein can be observed on the placenta. The needle is then used to puncture the placental vein and extract a tiny sample of blood through aspiration The sample should contain nearly pure fetal blood.

Obviously, the fetoscope was a sensible approach, and Dr. Frederic Frigoletto, our colleague in obstetrics, began to prepare himself to use it. With the instrument available to him, he first ascertained that he could safely obtain a blood sample from the fetus of a pregnant dog. Then he was prepared to try the instrument in human pregnancy. However, a powerful ethical issue stood in the way of direct application of the approach in an actual at-risk pregnancy. Until Frigoletto could satisfy himself that he could obtain a sample without fetal injury, he could not in good faith approach a pregnant woman with thalassemia trait who wished to have a prenatal diagnosis on her fetus. He could not do that unless he could give the woman his assurances that the procedure itself had a very low risk of causing the very abortion that the woman hoped to avoid.

There was only one way for Frigoletto to gain the necessary experience. He would have to ask normal pregnant women who, for their own personal reasons, had firmly decided to have an abortion to allow him to acquire a fetal blood sample the day before the abortion procedure. If he could do that several times, and if none of the fetuses actually aborted before the formal abortion procedure was performed, he would be fairly confident that the method was safe enough to apply in a pregnancy where the risk was having an infant with severe thalassemia.

We all agreed on the procedure to be followed. Frigoletto would obtain the practice samples as he had outlined; we would measure globin synthesis rates in them, and we would do enough of these practice cases to be sure that we could deliver a safe and reliable answer before we let it be known that we were ready to proceed in an actual case.

The next day, the *Boston Globe,* in a front-page story, reported that the proposed Massachusetts Fetal Research Law had gone through an important legislative committee and was about to be placed on the floor of the Massachusetts House of Representatives. The proposed law contained staggering statements. In brief, it would be a crime punishable by imprisonment for anyone to use fetal tissue for any research purpose whatsoever, nor would it be permissible to do any maneuvers prior to abortion and then examine the fetus to determine the results of those maneuvers. The law would shut down every possible type of fetal and even placental research in Massachusetts, and there would be no exceptions.

Harvard Medical School woke up to this news with surprise. The school had not been watching the legislature very carefully, and this development hit the entire scientific community like a thunderbolt. The young representative who had introduced the bill and the Speaker of the House, a wily old-time politico, were besieged with important medical figures who pointed out how much research would be injured. A strong argument was made by virologists, who pointed out that many viruses grow best on a framework of fetal cells; this law would have prevented the development of the polio vaccine. The authors of the bill, though firmly in the clutches of the right-to-life groups, were very intelligent men. They had not really appreciated how much they were doing to set back medical research. They were simply trying to write a law that would have stopped the antibiotic research study that had been performed at Boston City Hospital. They didn't want to stop everything.

In a series of endless meetings, we were able to chip away at the bill, but when the compromises were finally made, the fetoscope was still off limits. We could apply it all we wanted in a pregnancy at risk, but we could not test it first for safety in a pregnancy that was slated for abortion! I could see that this absurd conclusion bothered the authors of the bill tremendously. They wanted to find a way out of it, and they assured me that they *would* find a way out in a future modification, but the bill passed and Frigoletto could not acquire the experience that he believed he needed if he was ethically to offer the procedure to a pregnant woman who would count on the result.

I've many times asked myself why the authors of the bill, the young representative and the law professor, ever allowed themselves to get into such a box in the first place. Both were thoughtful and entirely decent men. Neither would wish to see a medical procedure put into practice without exhaustive safety checks. But the philosophical concept that no good should come from an evil act dominated their thinking when they wrote the law. Furthermore, they could not tolerate the notion that a human fetus should ever become the subject of biomedical testing no matter what the benefits to society might be. The entire focus of medicine should, in their opinion, be directed toward preserving the health of the fetus, even if the fetus was to be legally aborted in the next few hours.

It was part of the slippery slope Thomist argument that is used by some of the finest people I know. Oftentimes in our discussions, the history of the unspeakable Nazi-physician experiments on Jews and other minorities was recalled. If the helpless fetus was considered to be just another piece of tissue, the same sorts of hideous acts, if proposed by researchers to a mother who had no interest in the protection of her fetus, could be committed. The very actions would dehumanize the perpetrators and turn physicians into monsters.

I heard it all and I sympathized with much of it, but I kept returning to a simple principle. The fetus of a woman who is desperate to have her baby should have priority over the fetus of a woman who wants to abort. It is not immoral to ask women who are determined to end their pregnancies if they would be willing to help physicians learn how to save the fetuses of women who want to give birth.

The arguments and heated discussions went on for months. There were reams of position papers and unbelievably frequent drafts of new proposals. I learned firsthand how lawyers haggle over words. While all of this went on, a chill descended on fetal research in Boston. Uncertain about the law's interpretation, cautious hospital attorneys quietly advised their clients to abandon the field and move into something else. They were fearful that their clients would get bad press or, worse, end up with a prison sentence in Suffolk County, where the district attorney remained poised for another attack on the academic institutions.

I suppose it was the conservative opinion of the hospital lawyers more than any other issue that disturbed the authors of the bill. They did not want to chill all reasonable fetal research. They just didn't want it to be tied to abortion. They approved of our investigation into prenatal diagnosis of thalassemia and were trying to find language that would permit it. Indeed, they were strongly motivated by their own belief in the right of a pregnant woman to know everything she wishes to know about the health of her fetus. If her knowledge led to abortion, that was a sad result, but they strongly believed in the woman's right to know and make an informed decision. Thus they labored on, trying to find language that would preserve essential maternal rights while protecting the health of the fetus right up to its last moment of life.

Though the debates were fascinating and thrust me into the national discussions that had been launched by the actions of the Nixon administration, they were not advancing the prenatal diagnosis of thalassemia. Seeing that we would not rapidly develop the needed technology in Massachusetts, I decided to collaborate with John Hobbins and John Mahoney at Yale. They had just perfected their skills with the fetoscope and were ready to use it. With Henry Chang, a young research fellow in the laboratory and now at the United States Naval Hospital in Bethesda, we performed the first studies of human fetal globin chain synthesis, using the fetoscope to obtain the samples.

Y. W. Kan, now in San Francisco, was also hard at work on the problem. Collaborating with an obstetrician who used direct placental puncture, rather than a fetoscope, to obtain his samples, Kan performed the first prenatal diagnosis of homozygous beta thalassemia—that is, thalassemia caused by two defective beta globin genes. Shortly thereafter, with Blanche Alter leading our effort, we presented a series of fifteen prenatal diagnoses and clearly established that the fetoscope and our methods would be very useful in clinical practice.

The next step was the most important one of all. There are relatively few pregnancies at risk for beta thalassemia in the United States because the Italian and Greek communities are not rigidly self-contained here. Outbreeding, as the geneticists call it, is very common. Hence, the risk of marriage of two individuals with beta thalassemia trait is much lower in the United States than it is in more closed communities such as Sardinia, Cyprus, and mainland Greece. If we were to demonstrate that prenatal diagnosis is safe and accurate and that, when coupled with genetic counseling and selective abortion, it would actually reduce the incidence of beta thalassemia, we would have to transfer the technology as rapidly as possible to investigators in those countries.

Accordingly, Kan recruited Antonio Cao, the leading pediatric hematologist in Sardinia, where the incidence of beta thalassemia trait is as high as 30 percent of the population. Cao plunged into the effort there. Blanche Alter and I brought on board Dimitris Loukopoulos from Athens—also a skilled hematologist who had been trained by Phaedon Fessas. Loukopoulos took our methods back to Greece, where he persuaded the Greek army to undertake a population-wide screening program to detect thalassemia trait. All pregnant women with thalassemia trait giving birth in the major cities were offered prenatal diagnosis if their mates also had thalassemia trait.

Here were classical examples of practical expediency taking precedence over religious doctrine. The Catholic and Orthodox authorities chose to look the other way as these two men carried out an extraordinary effort to reduce the incidence of beta thalassemia in their communities through prenatal diagnosis, counseling, and selective abortion. The church authorities avoided the issue because they knew full well that the medical structure of the two communities could no longer stand the strain of the thalassemia caseload.

Had Sardinia and Greece been very undeveloped and impoverished, the burden of thalassemia on them would not have been as heavy because the new cases would not have been treated. They would certainly not have been transfused and treated with Desferal, and most children would have been left to die. In some remote communities, for example, babies with thalassemia are slowly starved to death. Italy and Greece, by contrast, have long traditions of medical support for the population, but the transfusion costs alone for thalassemia care were becoming prohibitive, and the amount of blood required had so strained the Sardinian and Greek blood banks that surgical schedules were often interrupted. Something had to be done to relieve the pressure. The church leaders knew it, and they decided to ignore what Cao and Loukopoulos were doing. While Bostonians were deciding whether to imprison Kenneth Edelin for performing a lawful abortion, the Italians and the Greeks were devoting their energies and emotions toward eliminating a centuries-old medical problem responsible for enormous suffering.

Today, the results of the efforts of those two physicians can only be called staggering. New cases of thalassemia have virtually disappeared from Sardinia and have been reduced to less than 10 percent of their former incidence in Greece. These examples of successful technology transfer and international cooperation remain extraordinary today. Cao and Loukopoulos deserve enormous credit for their undertaking.

Some years later, Blanche Alter established a registry of all of the prenatal diagnoses that had been performed with the fetoscope. To our great satisfaction, the diagnosis of two defective beta globin genes was made in 25 percent of the cases, exactly what one would predict if the method is accurate and if it is applied in enough cases to be statistically valid. The fetal loss rate was higher than we liked in the beginning of the experience as obstetricians gained skill. But losses rapidly declined to a level only slightly higher than that of amniocentesis, a standard technique. The fetoscope had been proven sufficiently safe. Mothers at risk of having babies with thalassemia could become pregnant without feeling that the outcome was entirely beyond their control.

Thus, a piece of clinical investigation that began when Bernie Forget entered our little laboratory at Children's Hospital with baby Maureen's blood smear turned out to have a profound influence on preventive medicine. Research grants from the National Institutes of Health and from private foundations such as the March of Dimes, the American Heart Association, and the American Cancer Society, and generous gifts from private individuals, supported fundamental research projects that led to international application of a successful preventive method. This is a gratifying example of the influence of fundamental and clinical research on disease prevention.

A few years after we developed our approach to prenatal diagnosis by fetal blood sampling, the new methods ushered in by the molecular biology revolution supplanted all of our techniques. Today, prenatal diagnosis of thalassemia can be carried out by studying the DNA in fetal skin cells obtained by amniocentesis or in samples of fetal cells snipped from the placenta. Only rarely are the fetoscope and fetal blood actually required. Had those molecular techniques been available in the early 1970s when the great Massachusetts fetal research fight was engaged, there would have been no issue to debate at all. This is an excellent example of how technology changes the nature of an ethical debate. The application of ethical principles is really quite fluid, changed by the technologic and social events that are in constant flux in a scientifically advancing society. Rigid adherence to a code of conduct that flies in the face of new facts must, in the end, fail. But the battles that ensue during the transitions can be damaging and demoralizing. I was fortunate to have the support of my colleagues and patients and of families like the Saifs. Without them, the struggle would have been lonely indeed.

The Recombinant
DNA Scare

AFTER DAYEM REPEATED his pledge to use the Desferal
pump and left the hospital for Washington on that fall day in
1981, I returned to the laboratory. Only among those lab benches
crowded with bright research fellows and graduate students, themselves surrounded by high-tech equipment and old-fashioned culture dishes, could I hope to conceive of an effective treatment for the
future. The excitement of discovery permeated the laboratory—new
information about genes was accumulating at an accelerating pace.

Watson and Crick had shown thirty years earlier that DNA is a
double helix made up of two complementary strands of nucleotide
bases (adenine, guanine, thymine, and cytosine), each linked to
sugar and phosphate molecules (figure 3). The discovery of the
structure of DNA immediately suggested a way for living cells to
pass their hereditary information on to daughter cells (through the
process called DNA replication). But it did not obviously point the
way to understanding how DNA, which consists of a linear string
of information, leads to the production (synthesis) of three-dimen-
sional proteins with a specific amino acid sequence.

Proteins are critical components in all aspects of growth and
metabolism. Each type of protein has a unique shape, with con-
tours, pockets, and folds that allow it to function in a specific way
(figure 4); insulin has a different shape from hemoglobin, the
albumin in plasma has a different shape from the myosin of muscle, and so on. The structural proteins are the most familiar to us;

they form muscle, elastic tissues, like tendons, and bones. But the set of proteins called enzymes are even more critical to living organisms, because they make things happen to otherwise static molecules. Enzymes do not themselves change the nature or direction of biochemical reactions, but their unique shape allows them to speed up and regulate all of the thousands of chemical reactions that allow bodies to function. Without enzymes, life processes would come to a grinding halt.

Figuring out how a string of As, Ts, Cs, and Gs in DNA could result in the production of specifically shaped proteins such as hemoglobin was high on everyone's list of important research topics in the late 1950s. In 1961 two groups of investigators, one headed by Sydney Brenner in England and the other by François Jacob in France, simultaneously reported a surprising finding: that the genes in DNA do not produce proteins directly but instead act through intermediaries. The process is illustrated in figure 8.

The first step in protein synthesis is the production of messenger RNA (mRNA). The process—called *transcription*—begins with the "unzipping" of the DNA molecule in the area of a particular gene. Next, certain enzymes in the nucleus grab hold of free-floating nucleotide bases and attach them to the gene in one strand of the unzipped DNA: an A is attached to every T in the gene, a C is attached to every G, and so on. All of the nucleotides in the chain are linked together. The resulting "copy" of the gene is actually not a true copy at all but more like the negative of a photograph: for every T in the DNA there is an A in the new chain, just as there is black instead of white in a negative. There is another important difference, however: wherever there was an A in the DNA, there is now a U instead of a T in the mRNA. Still, these single complementary chains of nucleotide bases look very much like the parent DNA except that they are much shorter and they contain ribose instead of deoxyribose as their sugar.

Each one of these new messenger RNA molecules corresponds to one gene. The chains of mRNA break away from the DNA as soon as they are formed, leave the nucleus, and enter the cell's cytoplasm—the part of the cell outside the nucleus. But messenger RNA is not itself a protein. Proteins are composed of amino acids,

The Genetic Control of Protein Synthesis: Transcription and Translation

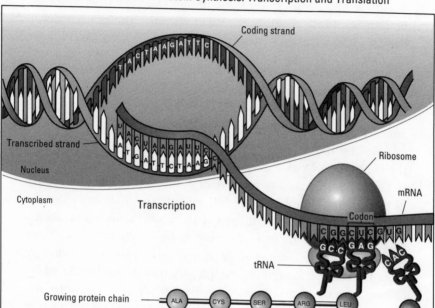

Figure 8 To make a protein molecule, the DNA double helix separates at the site of a gene, and transcribing enzymes (not shown) copy the bottom strand of nucleotides into a complementary mRNA strand. Where there is a G in the DNA, a C appears in mRNA; where there is a C in DNA, a G appears in mRNA; where there is a T, an A appears. However, an A in DNA appears as a U instead of a T in mRNA. Consequently, the upper or coding strand of the DNA has the same sequence as the mRNA except that T is present in DNA and U in mRNA. After the mRNA is transported from the nucleus, it joins ribosomes in the cytoplasm, where it is translated. Each codon (or triplet of bases) in the mRNA is complementary to a specific transfer RNA (tRNA), and each tRNA carries a specific amino acid to add to the growing protein chain. In this example, the amino acids arginine, leucine, and valine are being added to the chain, in the order dictated by the codons in the mRNA. When the chain is completed, it will fall off the mRNA-ribosome complex and become a functioning protein molecule.

not nucleotides. How does the encoded message transcribed in a nucleotide chain of mRNA become translated into a chain of amino acids?

Just as the stream of dots and dashes in Morse Code can only be translated into words by a skilled operator, the cell has developed a clever operation to read the code in mRNA. In 1961 we began to learn exactly how this genetic code works. Marshall Nirenberg at NIH proved that each amino acid is encoded by at least one triplet of bases called a *codon*. (For example, the amino acid arginine is encoded in mRNA by the sequence CGG, the amino acid leucine is encoded by the sequence CUC, and valine is encoded by the sequence GUG. These codons are represented in the genes in DNA as CGG, CTC, and GTG, respectively.) In 1966 H. Gobind Khorana, now a professor at the Massachusetts Institute of Technology, deciphered the entire *genetic code* defining all of the codons that call for each of the twenty amino acids that make up all proteins in the body. In the process he discovered that all but one of the twenty amino acids (methionine) can be encoded by more than one codon. (For example, arginine is also produced by five other codons, and leucine by five others as well.) Moreover, three codons (out of the total of sixty-four codons) do not specify any amino acid but rather cause protein production to stop altogether. These codons are therefore called "stop" codons; TAG in DNA is one example. In 1968 Nirenberg, Robert W. Holley, and Khorana received the Nobel Prize for their work in deciphering the genetic code.

The actual translation of the mRNA code into proteins occurs in complexes in the cytoplasm called *ribosomes*. In these microscopic assembly lines, special transfer RNAs (tRNAs) grab hold of free-floating amino acids and align each one with its corresponding three-base codon along the mRNA, according to the rules of the genetic code. The growing chain of amino acids that results is unique for every protein, and corresponds to the unique message contained in one gene. Hence the adage (coined by George Beadle in the 1940s), "One gene, one protein." In the mid-fifties and sixties, this information flow from DNA → RNA → protein became known as "the central dogma" of molecular biology.

Proteins can consist of hundreds of amino acids whose specific sequence determines how the protein will fold and shape itself and therefore how it will function in the body. Even one error in the sequence of an amino acid chain can cause the protein to fold incorrectly and therefore malfunction in the body, with sometimes serious consequences.

Sickle cell anemia illustrates how this kind of error works. The codon GAG (guanine-adenine-guanine) in DNA calls for the amino acid glutamic acid. That amino acid appears in the number 6 and number 39 positions of the beta chain in hemoglobin, and in many other positions in the chain as well. In a person who inherits sickle cell anemia, the beta globin gene contains a single mutation: the middle A of the number 6 codon, GAG, is changed (mutated) to a T. This *point mutation* produces the base triplet GTG, a codon for the amino acid valine when it appears as GUG in mRNA. So valine is present instead of glutamic acid in the number 6 position of the beta chain in sickle cell anemia. For reasons that are still not absolutely understood, that particular substitution of valine for glutamic acid at that site causes the hemoglobin molecule to elongate into a sickle form after the red cell has given up its oxygen to the body's tissues.

Because sickle cells are much more rigid than normal red cells, their passage through tiny capillaries is slow. The capillaries clog up with these slow-moving cells, and the result is periodic episodes of enormous pain. Chronic, progressive deterioration of various organs is also caused by the impaired circulation. The anemia associated with sickling red cells is brought on by their fragility and shortened life span. (Ironically, the anemia may itself protect against pain and organ degeneration to some degree, by lessening the number of red cells that can clog up the capillaries.)

Thus, inheriting one tiny substitution of one base for another in the genetic make-up can cause a person to become seriously ill. Most single base substitutions are harmless, but if they occur in a sensitive spot in the gene, a life-threatening inherited disease can be the consequence.

In the 1960s we did not yet know what kinds of base changes in codons could cause thalassemia. We did realize, however, that mRNA governs protein synthesis, and therefore we knew that the number of functioning beta mRNA molecules must be very large in normally developing red blood cells, and we surmised that they might be quite depressed in beta thalassemia. Our problem was that we didn't have the tools to measure globin mRNA production specifically, nor could we isolate the globin genes and determine why they might not be expressed in the form of mRNA.

To gain those tools, I decided to form an alliance of basic scientists and clinical investigators. In 1970, just as the molecular biology revolution was beginning to be applicable in medicine, our laboratory at Children's began a collaboration with Harvey Lodish, David Housman, and David Baltimore at the Massachusetts Institute of Technology. The two groups taught each other everything they could about their respective fields. Children's research and clinical fellows rubbed shoulders with MIT graduate students and postdoctoral fellows in the laboratories and in conference rooms. We shared data, planned experiments, and in the process committed ourselves to understanding the genetic details of pediatric blood diseases.

In our first collaborative experiments, Harvey Lodish, David Housman, and I quickly confirmed that the decoding machinery that produces beta hemoglobin chains from mRNA is normal in patients with thalassemia. In other words, the problem was not in the production or function of ribosomes, or transfer RNAs. Meanwhile, at Children's, Edward Benz (then a Harvard Medical student and now Chief of Medicine at the University of Pittsburgh) and Bernie Forget showed that the defect in thalassemia must be due to depressed messenger RNA activity. Other laboratories agreed with our findings, but the measurements were still indirect. We could not yet measure the number of globin mRNA molecules in a red cell.

A major breakthrough came as I was working on the problem with David Housman in Harvey Lodish's laboratory. Harvey shared the cramped lab space with David Baltimore, who was trained in virology and had spent several productive years examining the growth of polio virus and the enzymes it produces. He and the late Howard Temin of the University of Wisconsin were beginning to think about virology more broadly. Viruses that cause human disease are classified as either DNA viruses or RNA viruses, depending upon whether they contain a chromosome of either DNA or RNA surrounded by a protein coat. Viruses are cleverly adapted. They usually enter cells by fitting their protective coats into receptors on the cell surface. The receptors may have been designed for a different purpose, but the virus appropriates them. For example, HIV, the AIDS virus, has appropriated a vital immune cell receptor to gain entry into cells. Once inside, the tiny viral chromosome of nucleic acid directs the production of more viruses by using molecules stolen from the host cells. The newly produced viruses escape from the damaged host cell and invade new cells until their infectious replication is stopped by the body's immune response.

The life cycle of the standard DNA and RNA viruses was fairly well understood. It fit in very well with the central dogma of genetics, which clearly stated that DNA produces messenger RNA, which in turn produces proteins. But Temin and Baltimore were becoming very interested in another class of viruses called the RNA tumor viruses, which were thought to cause tumors only in animals.

The vexing problem facing Temin and Baltimore was this: how could an RNA virus cause unchecked proliferation of animal cells, since it didn't have any DNA to get the ball rolling? Could the viral RNA be transcribed *in reverse* into DNA, become incorporated into the host cell chromosome, and trigger a continuous growth signal? If so, they reasoned, there must be a special enzyme in the protein coat of these viruses, an enzyme that could convert RNA to DNA once the virus was inside the cell—a *reverse transcriptase*.

In their separate laboratories, the two investigators began to establish measurements that would detect the viral enzyme if it was there. Just as I walked into that crowded laboratory at MIT, the liquid scintillation counter was chattering away, printing radioactive counts on a paper strip. The Baltimore group had detected DNA production from RNA in a viral protein extract. Reverse transcriptase had been found! Howard Temin found it as well, and the two men received the Nobel Prize in 1975 for their discovery.

RNA tumor viruses are members of a type of viruses now referred to as *retroviruses*. In the early 1970s when Baltimore and

Temin discovered reverse transcriptase, retroviruses that infected humans were not known. Today human retroviruses occupy much of our attention because HIV (human immunodeficiency virus) which causes AIDS is a retrovirus.

My understanding of virology was, and still is, limited. I had my eyes on thalassemia and the production of hemoglobin. But reverse transcriptase looked like a way out of the box we were in as we struggled to find ways to measure globin mRNA. I immediately asked Baltimore whether reverse transcriptase could produce a DNA copy of globin mRNA. "Probably not," he said. "It's a viral enzyme, and it probably won't work on an animal or human RNA. But," and here he walked over to Inder Verma and Ron McCaffrey, postdoctoral fellows in his laboratory (Ron had had his clinical hematology training in my program at Children's), "Inder and Ron may want to take a crack at it if you can give them a decent mRNA sample from newly formed red cells." I explained to Verma and McCaffrey that Forget and Benz in my lab were very good at extracting mRNA from red cells, and they agreed to see whether reverse transcriptase would work on human globin mRNA.

The enzyme worked like a charm. In an immensely important collaboration, Verma, McCaffrey, Housman, Benz, Forget, and Baltimore added relatively well purified samples of beta globin mRNA to a tube containing viral reverse transcriptase and some other essential ingredients. Within moments they had a radioactive complementary copy of beta globin mRNA in their hands. They called it beta globin cDNA (the letter c standing for complementary because its base sequence is the precise opposite number of beta globin mRNA). They also produced radioactive alpha globin cDNA.

Armed with those radioactive cDNAs, Forget and the others moved swiftly to measure the number of beta and alpha mRNA molecules in normal and beta thalassemic red cells. In the samples they tested, including Dayem's cells, there were far fewer beta mRNAs than alpha mRNAs. Now we were homing in on the disease. At last we could say with confidence that most cases of beta thalassemia were due to the failure of beta mRNA to be exported from the nucleus to the decoding machinery of the cell.

The results of the probing of thalassemic cells with radioactive cDNA were exciting and clearly showed us that a new era of research was on the way, but we still had no great insight into the genetic basis of the disease. After all, our relatively old-fashioned studies had led us to a similar, if unproven, conclusion. We had shown several years before that beta globin production is deficient in beta thalassemia. It was satisfying to prove the concept, but we still did not know what was wrong with the beta globin genes in our patients. To acquire more sophisticated insight, we would have to wait for advances in technology that would permit us to examine the globin genes themselves. These advances were not long in coming.

WHILE Baltimore and Temin were attempting to understand reverse transcriptase, Hamilton Smith and Daniel Nathans at Johns Hopkins University were working on another set of bacterial enzymes which they called *restriction enzymes*. These proteins occur naturally in bacteria, serving as part of their defense system against the DNA of invading viruses. Viruses that invade bacteria are called *bacteriophages*, or *phages* for short. Restriction enzymes (so called because they restrict the range of bacterial hosts in which a virus can survive) attach themselves to the DNA of phages at specific sites and chop it into fragments, rendering the phage much less effective. Very quickly it was realized that the restriction enzymes discovered by Nathans and Smith could be used in the laboratory to chop up *any* large DNA molecule into smaller, more manageable pieces.

Restriction enzymes did not directly provide a base-by-base sequence of DNA, but they permitted analysis of the pattern and arrangement of the component pieces of that otherwise huge molecule. By analogy, we might think of the DNA molecule as a very long freight train. It's much easier to identify, count, and sequence the cars if the train is first stopped and then uncoupled at a few sites. Then the smaller groups of cars can be counted and the sequence of the cars readily established.

Since the work of Smith and Nathans (for which they also received the Nobel Prize), scores of restriction enzymes have been discovered, each with the capacity to cleave DNA at the site where a specific sequence of bases occurs, just as a train can be separated only at the couplers. By using several of these different enzymes, it soon became possible to slice DNA into ever smaller and more manageable pieces. When these individual pieces of double helix (now separated and rendered linear) are then placed in a semisolid matrix such as a gel and an electric current is passed through it, the different-sized fragments are separated according to their length. To detect a single DNA fragment containing a particular gene, one simply adds a molecule of radioactive cDNA made from the mRNA produced by that gene to the separated fragments. The cDNA attaches to the strand of DNA to which it is complementary. The radioactive signal serves as a probe, allowing the desired gene to be identified and even fished out of the matrix. This method is called a *Southern blot* after its inventor, Edward Southern, of the United Kingdom.

We started using some of these new techniques in the mid-1970s and began by asking two straightforward questions: Were beta and alpha mRNAs produced in the red cells of patients with beta or alpha thalassemia, and were beta and alpha globin genes present or absent in the DNA of those patients?

Y. W. Kan answered one of those questions. He had several Asian patients in San Francisco with different alpha thalassemia syndromes. Using a complex method by which he could measure mRNA in solution, he demonstrated a total absence of alpha globin mRNA in the young red cells of stillborn babies whose alpha globin genes were completely nonfunctioning. Similarly, Housman and Forget demonstrated a marked reduction of alpha mRNA molecules in a form of alpha thalassemia in which we were certain—but had not yet proven—that three of the four alpha genes are either missing or nonfunctioning. Shortly thereafter, Stuart Orkin in our laboratory examined the DNA of patients with alpha thalassemia using the then new Southern blot method. He confirmed that there is complete absence of alpha globin genes in babies who die of the disease at birth and also showed that the patients studied by Housman and Forget have one copy of the alpha gene remaining.

Our studies of alpha thalassemia and those of others taught us that entire deletions of alpha genes characterize most of the various forms of alpha thalassemia. But we were disappointed when we turned to beta thalassemia. In the vast majority of patients, including Dayem, there was no evidence of a beta gene deletion. We concluded that they must have point mutations in their beta genes—single base substitutions in the DNA that are impossible to find by the Southern blot method but which cause severe dysfunction or deficiency of beta mRNA. Before we could find those mutations, we had to await improved methods of DNA base sequencing.

In 1975 Fred Sanger of Cambridge, England, who had already received a Nobel Prize for his development of methods used in the analysis of the sequence of amino acids in proteins, created a very important approach to DNA base sequencing. An even more readily adaptable method was established in 1977 by Allan Maxam and Walter Gilbert of Harvard. Their technique was improved still further by Sanger, and today DNA base sequencing has become a routine procedure in laboratories around the world. The Nobel Prize was awarded to Sanger (his second) and Gilbert for these important contributions.

Once a method for sequencing genes was available, the next obvious requirement was to create enough copies of a globin gene to sequence it. Without sufficient copies, no method could detect the bases. But how could we cause specific genes to multiply in a test tube? The techniques that would make that possible form the basis of gene cloning and recombinant DNA methodology.

In the minds of some, the terms *recombinant DNA* and *gene cloning* conjure up threatening images of frightening, invasive organisms that might escape from some Dr. Frankenstein's laboratory and spread highly infectious diseases or virulent forms of cancer. What in fact is gene cloning and why does it suggest such dire consequences to the naive as well as some of the more sophisticated?

The idea that genes are made of DNA and that they might be isolated and cloned (that is, reproduced exactly) and then transferred to organisms was derived from Oswald Avery's studies of bacteria that began in the mid-1940s. He and his colleagues discovered that the formation of capsules (sugary coats) by pneumococci (the organisms that cause pneumonia) is controlled by genes, that the genes are present in the DNA of the pneumococci, and that incubation of non-capsule-forming pneumococci with the DNA of capsule-forming pneumococci would induce capsule formation. This was the first instance of gene therapy.

Soon thereafter, other investigators showed that *E. coli*, which live in everyone's gut, bear a single linear DNA chromosome. (In humans, by contrast, DNA is distributed among forty-six chromosomes.) The bacterial chromosome contains the genes that produce mRNAs, which in turn produce enzymes and other proteins.

But in addition to their primary chromosome, bacteria also carry circular pieces of DNA called *plasmids*. These contain genes that may be unique to the plasmid or may be present in exact copies within the bacterial chromosome. The genetic make-up of a plasmid is continually changing in nature, as it picks up whole genes or fragments of genes from the bacterial chromosome and from invading viruses. When a bacterium multiplies to form a clone, the plasmids within it also replicate and become part of both daughter cells, and any gene that happens to be part of the plasmid at the moment of replication will go along for the ride. This process goes on continuously in nature and is going on in the intestines of anyone who is reading this book. Given the rapid doubling of bacteria and plasmids, our guts are enormously efficient recombinant DNA, or gene-cloning, mills.

This ability of plasmids to change and multiply continuously is one of the major reasons that antibiotics sometimes lose their effectiveness. To understand how antibiotic resistance works, we must recall that commercial antibiotics are often based on processes that bacteria use in nature to protect themselves against other microbes. For example, bacteria have developed some enzymes that can cause holes to form in the cell walls of other bacteria, others that block DNA replication, or others that interfere with RNA synthesis, and still others that prevent protein chain elongation. Commercial antibiotics cause these same sorts of destruction.

But in the microbial world, as in the human world, warfare sometimes escalates, as bacteria evolve new weapons to resist those previously developed by their enemies. It turns out that the instructions for the production of these new weapons of resistance are often incorporated into the genes of plasmids. As bacteria and their associated plasmids replicate, the genes conferring resistance to the antibiotics of the enemy replicate as well. And as bacteria unfortunate enough not to carry the resistant plasmid succumb either to their natural enemies or to a commercial antibiotic, all that are left standing on the field are resistant bacteria. Drug resistance is, today, one of the most important barriers to the control of serious infectious diseases.

How do bacteria insert antibiotic resistance genes into plasmids? The answer is really quite simple, and all the work is done by enzymes. They produce certain restriction or DNA-cutting enzymes of the type described by Smith and Nathans to slice open a plasmid. Then other enzymes cause both ends of the opened circle of DNA to become "sticky"; still other enzymes create sticky ends on the ends of the resistance gene, which cause the piece of resistance gene to fit into the plasmid; and a final enzyme closes the circle. Now the resistance gene is neatly placed in the plasmid circle, ready to multiply.

If germs can do all of that cutting and splicing and replicating of selected genes, why couldn't scientists, armed with restriction enzymes and fragments of cDNA, do the same thing? That is, why couldn't they insert any gene of their choice—say, one taken from a plant or animal or human—and insert it into a plasmid (see figure 9) and just wait for the desired gene to replicate thousands of times? The answer, of course, is that they now can.

WHEN investigators at Stanford, headed by Paul Berg, proposed these new recombinant DNA techniques in 1971, the scientific world held its breath with anticipation, but the enthusiasm was not unbridled. There were a few cautious individuals, including Berg, who sounded some important warnings. Though the effete bacteria that are used to clone genes in the laboratory are certainly feeble on their own, would they become newly strength-

Cloning a Beta Globin Gene

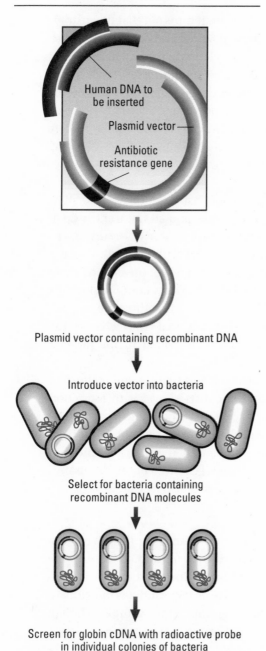

Human DNA to be inserted

Plasmid vector

Antibiotic resistance gene

Plasmid vector containing recombinant DNA

Introduce vector into bacteria

Select for bacteria containing recombinant DNA molecules

Screen for globin cDNA with radioactive probe in individual colonies of bacteria

Figure 9 Plasmids are double circles of DNA that enter and replicate in bacteria. To clone a beta globin gene, an antibiotic resistance gene is first inserted into a plasmid, and then a piece of human DNA containing a beta globin gene is inserted. The circle is closed, and the new recombinant plasmid is mixed with bacteria. It enters a few of them and confers antibiotic resistance to them. When all of the bacteria are exposed to an antibiotic, only those that contain the plasmid with the antibiotic resistance gene (as well as the globin gene that went along for the ride) survive. Therefore, all the remaining bacteria contain a beta globin gene. The bacteria can be grown to very high numbers and the beta globin DNA purified from them.

ened if they were fortified with the cDNAs prepared from human or animal cells? Would they be able to leap out of their incubators and act like an Andromeda strain? What if tumor genes were to be inserted into them? Would cancer become an epidemic infectious disease?

A historic conference designed to discuss the risks and benefits of the new technology was held in Asilomar, California, in February 1975. It began with an introduction to the problem by David Baltimore and included remarks by many of the leaders of the field. An important summary of the conference called for careful and controlled experiments and close collaboration between experts in recombinant DNA research and experts in bacteriology and virology. It was a far-sighted and thoughtful document that encouraged the research but called for careful management and safety standards.

In 1976 the National Institutes of Health responded by forming its Recombinant DNA Advisory Committee. The RAC was created to establish appropriate and safe standards and to review specific applications for individual experiments. That in itself created an enormous slowdown as the applications began to pile up. Bureaucracy was now the leading consumer of the recombinant DNA revolution. Many scientists expressed their concern that important experiments of great value to biology and medicine were being needlessly delayed. Others felt that ample time was needed to establish the correct procedures. We had to know, they thought, whether expensive containment facilities would be required. If so, for what kinds of experiments would they be necessary? If the public was to be reassured, they argued, we would have to be cautious and move with very deliberate speed.

As is often the case in science, there was a small group of investigators, including some with excellent reputations, who voiced almost hysterical concern. They formed a vociferous minority determined to block or delay as long as possible the successful application of this technology in biology and medicine. As might be predicted, this group's motives and beliefs were heterogeneous. Some were sincerely concerned about the health hazards and had no personal motivations other than their profound worries about the public's health. These were very rare individuals, because the health hazards were very difficult to define in any realistic fashion.

Another small group represented those who felt left behind. They were scientists who had had important roles in another era and saw that they were about to leave the center stage to become bit players. Their feelings were understandable, but their behavior was inexcusable. They were loud champions of delay and obfuscation.

A third group was particularly pernicious. They were the children of the dark Vietnam War days of the 1970s. They saw themselves as liberals, and viewed genetic research as a terrible threat to individual rights and as a tool of racism. In their zeal to oppose any hint of biological (as opposed to environmental) determinism, they fought against the new science because they feared the information it might produce. This was the period that immediately followed the Civil Rights revolution in the United States and was also the period during which a largely black United States army fought the most unpopular war in U.S. history, while a largely white, highly educated, and very "liberal" group remained at home and protested in the streets. Richard Nixon presided over this nasty stew, an odorous pot that boiled over in nearly every corner of American society. In their understandable hostility to anything that smacked of racism, these protesting scientists sometimes lost control of their own scientific judgment.

Accompanying the battle over the entrance of recombinant DNA science at Harvard were two additional examples of the unfortunate behavior of this small group. In 1975 a thoughtful entomologist on the Cambridge campus named Edward Wilson wrote a remarkable book entitled *Sociobiology*. In it he reviewed the social behavior of a wide range of insects and other animals and pointed out that many aspects of insect behavior must be genetically determined. He suggested in addition that the social behavior of higher organisms might also have a genetic component. The book is a masterpiece of scholarship, but it was greeted by a handful of Wilson's colleagues as an example of neoracism and biological determinism. Students were encouraged by these colleagues to boycott Wilson's classes, demonstrate in front of his home, and interrupt him at lectures. Their rudeness and their open abuse of academic freedom was frightening to behold. In a certain sense, these students and the faculty members who encouraged them were saying, "We are liberals, and if you aren't a liberal exactly like us, we will destroy you." In their zeal to be politically correct, they threw away the norms of university behavior and acted like the very bullies they so despised in the public sector.

In another example, this time in Harvard Medical School, Park Gerald, who had described very important abnormal hemoglobins, and Stanley Walzer, a colleague in psychiatry, had made an interesting observation about the sex chromosomes in some males. Gerald had become an expert in a field called cytogenetics. He could examine preparations of human chromosomes, tell them all apart, and diagnose many inherited diseases from abnormalities of their shape and size. He and Walzer proposed that individuals with a rare anomaly in which males have two Y (male) chromosomes and an X (female) chromosome—instead of one Y and one X, as in normal males—might exhibit more violent (androgenic) behavior than usual. In fact, the anomaly seemed to be found at a higher than expected frequency among prison inmates. When the two published their findings, their so-called liberal colleagues took to the streets. There were shouting matches, demonstrations, and threats of violence. Gerald and Walzer, they argued, were ascribing behavior to inheritance as well as to environment, an unforgivable sin. (The truth is that the sample size was too small to draw firm conclusions one way or the other.)

In this setting of social, academic, and racial conflict, Harvard University proposed to construct a new laboratory for recombinant DNA research that would contain the safety features demanded by the NIH-sponsored Recombinant DNA Advisory Committee. The Massachusetts Institute of Technology also announced plans to build such a facility. It was 1976, the year of the nation's bicentennial celebration and the first year of a new Democratic administration in Washington. But all was not bright in Cambridge, Massachusetts, at least not for Harvard University or MIT. As soon as the plans for the new laboratory were announced, a small group of faculty members from both institutions allied themselves with some community activists to oppose the plan.

Nothing could have given certain Cambridge politicians, particularly its mayor, more pleasure than the scene that played out before them. Here were the great, proud, and non-tax-paying Harvard and MIT, the favorite targets of the ordinary Cambridge politician, beseeching the Cambridge City Council to grant building permits. And here were some faculty members denouncing their own institutions as cold-blooded giants ready to sacrifice the health of the defenseless Cambridge citizenry for the evil pelf that the institutions would earn from research grants. What a delectable moment for a pol whose only substantial contribution to Cambridge life was the fixing of traffic tickets for loyal supporters.

I will never forget the scene in the packed Council chambers on that hot August night. The room was filled with a dense cloud of obfuscation and the sweat of overheated bodies. The more sensible councilors quickly saw that nothing was to be gained from such a circus, and the mayor, after having had his moment as the ringmaster, reluctantly agreed to request the city manager to appoint a commission of citizens to listen to both sides of the debate and come up with recommendations. Soon thereafter, the proceedings began.

I was very much part of those hearings because I became convinced that recombinant DNA research would open up possibilities for all of my patients with thalassemia that were hitherto impossible to achieve. I could see the future of simplified prenatal diagnosis conducted without any risk to the fetus, and I could even envisage the creation and insertion of a normal beta globin gene into young patients with beta thalassemia, to cure their illness once and for all. When an opponent spoke of the near sacredness of present strains of bacteria and the sin of changing them, I replied that bacteria are changing themselves all the time. Furthermore, I told the committee that I don't conduct a love affair with germs. Some of them are quite nasty and hurt my patients very badly.

In the end, the commission, some of whom were my neighbors, voted to allow Harvard to construct the new laboratory and to permit MIT to remodel suitable space as well. That vote opened the doors to DNA research at Harvard and MIT. As a result, Dayem's disease began to receive a huge new infusion of effort.

Failing Genes

B Y 1980, using the many new methods of recombinant DNA technology, researchers in inherited blood diseases had sequenced the bases in all of the normal hemoglobin genes. That huge advance led, in turn, to the complete molecular description of the many different thalassemia genes, including those causing Dayem's particular illness. The rather surprising model of the globin genes that eventually emerged proved considerably more complex than had been expected.

Important advances in understanding the complex structure of *all* genes occurred in the mid-1970s with a discovery made by Philip Sharp at MIT. While studying the DNA of viruses, Sharp found that their gene structure is analogous to a long freight train that contains several loaded cars interspersed by many empty ones. As messenger RNA is transcribed from DNA, the empty cars are cut out and pushed away from the mRNA, while the loaded ones are connected together. The new train of mRNA is much shorter than the gene itself, but every car contains an important load of information about the protein it is programmed to produce. For that discovery, Sharp received a share of the 1993 Nobel Prize.

A few months after Sharp's publication, Philip Leder, then at the National Institutes of Health and now chairman of the Department of Genetics at Harvard Medical School, reported that human globin genes have the same peculiar structure as viral genes. The beta globin gene, for example, is not a solid block of DNA base se-

The Beta Globin Gene and the Production of Beta Globin

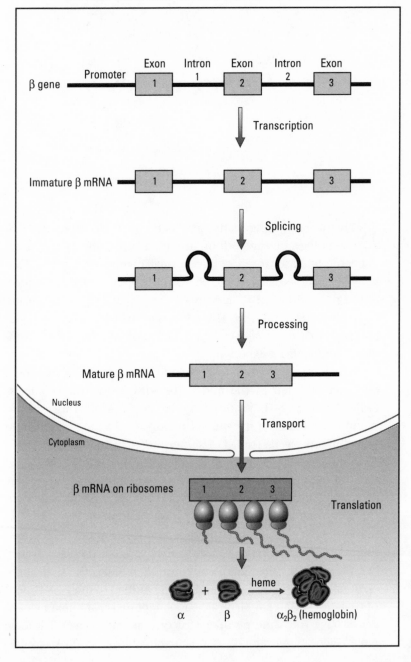

quences that form the base triplets or codons for beta globin mRNA. Instead, there are three different and widely separated coding blocks of base triplets in the gene. The coding blocks are called *exons*. The exons are interrupted by two different intervening sequences of noncoding bases, called *introns*. Why the introns are present or why they are located between the exons is known only to evolution, but they occur in all globin genes and in almost all other mammalian genes as well. They may have something to do with gene or mRNA stability, but we still do not know exactly why they are present or what functions they serve. In any case, if one were to seize a pair of molecular scissors and cut both of the complementary strands of the beta globin gene out of their resting places on chromosome 11, they would look like the structure at the top of figure 10.

In the genes of all organisms, there are still other sequences in the DNA that control the rate at which the so-called structural genes are expressed. As early as the 1940s, the American geneticist Barbara McClintock, working with maize, discovered a number of these "controlling elements," some of which seemed to move unpredictably from location to location on the chromosome! She began to publish papers about inhibitors, inducers, and other regulatory sequences of DNA, but her work was largely ignored. Many of her ideas were thought to be bizarre, especially those jumping genes.

Meanwhile, in Paris, François Jacob and Jacques Monod began to wonder how cells turn on or off their production of a given protein just as needed. Cells have many more genes than they express at any given time. In fact, if they were to continuously express all their genes, the result would be chaos. Soon Jacob and

Figure 10 The beta globin gene (and all human globin genes) has two introns and three exons. Following transcription into immature mRNA, the introns are "looped out" (excised) and the exons are spliced together. Next, the ends of the mRNA are altered (processed) to produce mature mRNA. The mRNA molecule is then transported from the nucleus to the ribosomes, where it is translated into beta globin chains. These combine with alpha globin chains and heme to produce adult hemoglobin.

Monod began to identify some of the mechanisms in DNA respon-sible for regulating gene expression. Many of these involved the production of enzymes that themselves activate other genes. Words like *operator, repressor,* and *enhancer* began to enter the everyday vocabulary of people working on the regulation of gene expression. In 1983, half a century after her contributions were first published, McClintock's prescient work in this area was recognized with a Nobel Prize.

Soon it was determined that at the beginning of globin genes (and in other genes as well), a sequence of bases called a *promoter* regulates the rate at which the gene produces messenger RNA (see figure 10). Given all of this complexity in the structure and func-tion of globin genes, it's little wonder that plenty of opportunities arise for genetic mistakes. We began to realize that unlike sickle cell anemia, thalassemia was likely to have several causes. Immediately after the normal globin gene sequences were understood, two lines of thalassemia research began. First, we had to know the locations or maps of all of the globin genes. And second, we had to find the disturbances in those maps that cause the many different thalas-semia syndromes. Between 1975 and 1985 scientists working in several laboratories completely defined the maps of the beta and alpha globin gene clusters and the precise base sequences of the genes on chromosomes 11 and 16 respectively. The map of the beta gene cluster is shown in figure 11. The beta cluster is actually a series of related genes that occupies about 40,000 bases (40 kilo-bases; 40kb) of DNA on chromosome 11.

The cluster begins on the left with a gene called epsilon (ε). It is a beta-like gene that is expressed only very early in fetal develop-ment. It is then switched off and is followed both anatomically as well as functionally by the two gamma genes, one called G gamma (Gγ) and the other A gamma (Aγ). These two genes are nearly identical and are expressed with the alpha genes on chromosome 16 to produce the fetal hemoglobin that is present in the rest of fetal life. The gamma genes are followed by a delta gene. This gene has many features of a beta gene, but it has a different base se-quence that causes it to function at a very low level. It is therefore an unimportant gene. The final gene in the cluster is the vital beta gene itself. Its function replaces that of gamma genes when the fetus is nearly ready for birth. That process of replacement is called the fetal switch (see figure 6 on page 32). A similar map of the alpha gene cluster was also constructed.

When the maps of the beta and alpha gene clusters had been established, we next needed to know the fine structure of the individual genes. What were the normal base sequences of the alpha, gamma, and beta genes, and what were the various mutations in those sequences that could disrupt their function and cause thalassemia, a failure of sufficient globin chain production? We owe the information about normal globin genes to many laboratories around the world, but all agree that Tom Maniatis, now a professor of biochemistry and molecular genetics at Harvard, was a major

Map of the Beta Cluster on Chromosome 11 and Some Beta Gene Deletions

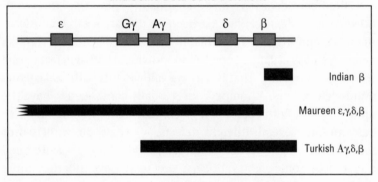

Figure 11 The beta-like globin genes are arranged on chromosome 11 in the order of their transcription during development. The epsilon gene is transcribed in embryonic life, the two gamma genes in fetal life, and the beta gene in adult life. (The delta gene is a low output gene and therefore unimportant.) Three of the many deletions that cause beta zero thalassemia are shown here. In India, a common, small deletion affects the "downstream" half of the beta gene. In baby Maureen, the epsilon gene, both gamma genes, the delta gene, and the "upstream" half of the beta gene were deleted. The deletion extends upstream well beyond the epsilon gene, to a point that has not been precisely determined. In the Turkish baby, for whom prenatal diagnosis using DNA was first attempted, a large deletion involving the A gamma, delta, and beta genes was mapped.

leader in the effort. Others, including Sherman Weissman of Yale University's Department of Genetics, were very important contributors as well. The international collaborative effort that accompanied the research was extraordinary because everyone with any knowledge of the scientific revolution then in progress knew that the information about the hemoglobin genes that we were about to gain would be widely applied in all of the biomedical sciences. The stakes were enormous for basic science and particularly for medicine.

As we considered the molecular basis of beta thalassemia, we had to confront the fact that the errors in beta thalassemia genes differ in severity. Some of the genes, called *beta zero* thalassemia genes, produce no beta globin chains at all. Others, called beta plus genes, like Dayem's, markedly reduce but do not entirely abolish beta globin chain production. The simplest cause of a beta zero defect would be a complete or even a partial gene deletion. The cause of a beta plus defect was, at first, more difficult to imagine.

These considerations made abundantly clear that the words *heterozygote* and *homozygote,* particularly the latter, can be misleading when applied to thalassemia. In reference to genetic diseases, a heterozygote is usually defined as an individual with a defect in one copy of a given gene. That is why we call patients with thalassemia trait heterozygotes. A homozygote is usually considered to have the same defect in both copies of a given gene. Since thalassemia may be caused by several different defects, many people with two or more defects might best be called *compound* or *mixed heterozygotes,* rather than homozygotes, because they may have inherited more than one kind of mutation, a different one from each parent. That proved to be the case with Dayem.

The first approach to mapping beta thalassemia genes was to use the Southern blot method and various restriction enzymes and radioactive cDNA probes to search for large deletions of the beta genes that might cause the disease. This had been a very profitable approach in the alpha thalassemias because it turned out that alpha gene deletion is a common cause of alpha thalassemia, at least in Asians. But the method was singularly unrevealing in most cases of either beta zero or beta plus thalassemia. Very few cases were due to deletions—at least to deletions large enough to be detected by the Southern approach. There were important exceptions, however, and a vital opportunity to detect such a deletion arose in the first application of molecular biology to the prenatal diagnosis of thalassemia.

Cigdem Altay is a pediatric hematologist at Hacettepe University in Turkey who came to Children's Hospital for fellowship training in genetics in 1966, the year that I transferred my laboratory from the Brigham Hospital to Children's. She returned to Turkey to be a faculty member and a consultant in hematology, where she kept abreast of our efforts in prenatal diagnosis, knowing that the technology would be important in her country.

Thalassemia is a critical public health problem in Turkey. In 1978 a Turkish woman in the early stages of pregnancy came to see Altay. The woman was accompanied by Susan Griffey, an American nurse who was then working in a health clinic in the small Turkish town where the patient lived. The story was a familiar one. Her first child had died of thalassemia at the age of three during an episode of infection. Could Altay tell her whether the present fetus was also affected? Altay could not, but she asked the patient whether she would be willing to travel to Boston, where she knew that Blanche Alter and I were trying to develop a prenatal diagnostic system using the fetoscope and fetal vein sampling.

Altay also investigated the hemoglobin genetics in the family. Both the woman and her husband were carriers of a rare form of thalassemia. They both had small red cells and mild anemia just like ordinary people with beta thalassemia trait. But here the resemblance stopped. Unlike most trait carriers, they had strikingly high levels of fetal hemoglobin. It was apparent that both of these parents had what is called delta-beta thalassemia trait, a complete loss of function (and probably a deletion) of both the delta and beta genes in the beta cluster on one copy of chromosome 11. In that condition, the gamma genes to the left of the deletion seem to function at a higher than normal rate. Usually, people who are homozygous for this condition have rather mild anemia; their course may be very much like that of Mr. Zhanghi, who undoubtedly had a delta-beta thalassemia gene and a relatively mild beta plus thalassemia gene.

Altay informed the expectant mother and father that their next child should have mild thalassemia even if he or she inherited the abnormal chromosome 11 from each parent. But the parents, having already lost one child to thalassemia, were vehement in their request for prenatal diagnosis. They did not wish to give birth to another child with this life-threatening disease. To help the family and to learn more about thalassemia and its prenatal diagnosis, Susan Griffey accompanied the prospective parents to Boston, where, in her excellent Turkish, she could act as translator and interpret our findings and opinions to them.

We set to work as soon as the family arrived. Here, we believed, was a unique opportunity. If the parents each had a deletion of delta and beta genes on one copy of their two beta clusters, Stuart Orkin might be able to determine this by performing a Southern blot analysis and probing with a radioactive beta cDNA. If equal amounts of DNA were applied to the gel, the beta gene band in the parents should have about half of the radioactivity of the band that would be produced by the DNA of a normal individual. Such a finding would be very dependent on careful DNA loading and therefore somewhat unreliable—it would not be a proof of the deletion. But it would encourage us to believe that we could detect a fetus who had inherited two delta-beta deletions because in that condition there would be no radioactive beta band at all.

The results were indeed encouraging. The beta band identified in the parents' Southern blot had about half of the radioactivity as the same band derived from several normal individuals. We were confident that if we could obtain a sample of the fetus's DNA, we could determine whether the fetus was a homozygote (having two deletions) or a normal (having no deletions)—there was a 25 percent chance of either—or was a heterozygote like its parents (having one deletion and one normal gene). The fetus had a 50 percent chance of the latter.

Since neither we nor anyone else had ever tried to perform a prenatal diagnosis using fetal DNA and the Southern blot method, we took no chances. We sent the patient with Susan Griffey to our colleagues in New Haven, where Dr. John Hobbins used the fetoscope to obtain a sample of fetal blood as well as a sample of the fetal skin cells that float in the amniotic fluid. We set aside the fetal skin cells in a tissue culture flask and prayed that they would multiply enough for us to probe them for their beta gene content. Meanwhile, we performed the standard study of the fetal blood with a radioactive amino acid to determine whether we could observe any production of beta globin in the fetal red cells; the next day, with bated breath, we analyzed the results.

To our delight, there was about half the usual production of beta globin in the red cells of the fetus, the same levels we had found in the parents' red cells. Clearly this fetus was not in danger. It had thalassemia trait like its parents and would be a healthy baby. We told the parents what we believed to be the good news, and their reaction was wonderful to behold. They literally screamed with relief and hugged and kissed us. Then they wrapped their arms around Griffey and hugged her until she couldn't breathe. It was one of the happiest moments in my medical career. We had a marvelous celebration at Sue Griffey's home, just before she and the family returned to Turkey. A huge Turkish meal was prepared with ingredients scoured from the ethnic shops of Boston. A few months later, a healthy child with thalassemia trait was born.

A few weeks after this positive blood test result, the fetal cells we were culturing had grown to sufficient numbers to permit Stuart Orkin to probe them in a Southern analysis. Again the radioactivity was half of normal, confirming the analysis we had performed on the fetal blood. A few months later, however, Orkin defined the limits of the beta cluster deletion in this family and found that it was larger than we thought. It encompassed the beta gene, the delta gene, and the A gamma gene as well. If the baby had been a homozygote and if the mother had chosen not to abort, her child might have had more severe disease than we originally thought.

This case was the first application of modern molecular technology in prenatal diagnosis and ushered in an entirely new era of this methodology. It was also one of the first attempts to define a beta gene deletion by molecular probing. Today, fetal blood sampling is almost entirely a technique of the past, having been replaced by molecular probing of fetal skin or placental cells.

THE NEXT attempt to define the molecular basis of beta thalassemia came from a suggestion by David Weatherall, the leader of the Oxford thalassemia group. He knew of our experience with the Turkish baby and hoped Orkin would have a look at one of his Indian patients with beta zero thalassemia. Weatherall's uncanny judgment about what might be a productive scientific venture proved right again when Orkin discovered a deletion in the far right-hand portion of the man's beta gene. Today we know that this particular deletion is present in as much as 30 percent of the cases of beta thalassemia in India.

In the same year, Sergio Ottolenghi and his colleagues in Italy demonstrated that certain Italians with beta zero thalassemia and relatively high levels of fetal hemoglobin have large deletions in both chromosomes that encompass the beta and the delta gene. Not long after, Orkin defined the very large deletion that we knew must be present in Maureen, the baby with gamma-delta-beta thalassemia. Dorothy Tuan, Sherman Weissman, and Bernie Forget, all at Yale, and Arthur Bank at Columbia soon described intermediate-sized deletions that we now call delta-beta thalassemia or hereditary persistence of fetal hemoglobin (HPFH). These unusual mutations are all causes of beta zero thalassemia because all or part of the beta gene is deleted. They vary in their severity, depending upon the amount of residual gamma chain production that remains. I'm sure that one of Mr. Zhanghi's thalassemia genes must have been of this type. For reasons that are still not entirely understood, a great deal of gamma chain production may ensue if a delta and beta gene deletion occurs and both gamma genes remain intact.

As revealing as all of these cases were, we soon had to concede that large deletions represent a very minor fraction of the beta thalassemia mutations, even among the beta zero thalassemias. The vast majority of the beta thalassemias are due to much smaller point mutations that cannot be detected by the relatively simple Southern blot analysis. The first major step toward the definition of the small point mutations was made by Y. W. Kan. Ever since he arrived in San Francisco, he had wondered about the dogma that most of us then believed: that the problem in beta thalassemia must always be a failure in the production of beta messenger RNA in the nucleus and therefore an insufficiency of beta mRNA in the cell where beta globin chains are produced.

As soon as Kan established his laboratory at the San Francisco County General Hospital, he began to probe with radioactive beta cDNA the red cells of his beta thalassemic patients. Many of them were Chinese because the members of the Bay Area Chinese community tend to use that hospital for their medical care, and Kan could communicate with them very readily. Quite soon after Kan began working, he phoned me to express concern that he could not exactly confirm the results that Forget and Housman were finding. They had maintained that they could find almost no beta mRNA in their nondeletion beta zero patients, whereas Kan, while observing some reduction of beta mRNA in a Chinese patient, was certain that the deficiency was more moderate than severe.

The difference was crucial, and we both knew it. Forget and Housman were saying that nondeletional beta thalassemia was due to near failure to produce any beta mRNA, while Kan was suggesting that such patients might actually make beta mRNA but that the mRNA did not function. Later on, we realized that both sets of laboratories were quite correct, but at the time we thought that beta thalassemia occurred in only a few ways. We had no idea that there are many different nondeletional mutations that cause the disease. We were looking for one or two master causes, not many.

As Kan and I talked, it became clear that his major concern was that he might be making a technical error. After all, the methods were new, and he was on his own for the first time. I was much less concerned about that possibility. He has excellent hands in the laboratory. I doubted error and began to wonder about the likelihood of important differences among ethnic groups. I was in an awkward position, however. Bernie Forget was then a valued member of a research laboratory of which I was the leader. He was collaborating with David Housman of MIT. Kan had established his own independent laboratory in San Francisco and was beginning to compete with Forget and Housman and the others in my group. I had worked happily and productively with Kan for many years and yearned for his success. How could I be loyal to both sides?

There was only one way to deal with the problem. I decided that I would never tell Forget and Housman what Kan was doing, and I would never give any information to Kan about the findings of Forget and Housman. This would not be easy because I was privy to everything that both sets of laboratories were doing. My concern was that I would slip and tell something to someone without recognizing the source of my information. Fortunately, I was sufficiently careful and did not slip up. The two groups competed in a friendly and entirely honorable way, and I was able to keep my excellent relationship with both of them.

Well-respected researchers like Kan, Forget, and Housman, though highly competitive, play by the rules of the game, which include a willingness to share important information with others upon a firm understanding that the shared data will not be released without the approval of all concerned, a respect for confidentiality, and a citation of the important contributions of competitors. Yet competition in science is often criticized in the press and even in some academic circles because there are well-publicized cases of unsavory behavior, particularly by large laboratories that are racing to achieve an important goal. Lost in the polemics over appropriate behavior may be the simple fact that competition is the vital engine of science. Absent their striving for recognition, grants from public and private foundations, promotion, and higher income, most scientists would relax in a tweedy academic atmosphere and progress would slow to a crawl. The blunt truth is that the driving force of scientific progress is the struggle by thousands of scientists to find room at the top of their profession, where laboratory support is assured for only a small fraction of the competitors.

Since Kan had strong reason to believe that there was something wrong with the beta mRNA in his Chinese patient with beta zero thalassemia, he decided to examine the mRNA very carefully. To do so, he made a cDNA with reverse transcriptase, and sequenced the bases. To his delight, he found a single base substitution at codon 17, where the AAG for lysine was changed to the "stop" codon TAG. This kind of mutation is called a *nonsense mutation*. When an mRNA carrying it enters the cytoplasm for translation on the ribosomes, it acts like a crippled molecule.

Whenever a ribosome comes to a nonsense mutation, all protein chain elongation ceases and the ribosome falls away. The shortened piece of protein is degraded by other enzymes in the cytoplasm. In this case, every time a ribosome moved to the stop codon 17, translation of beta globin would cease, and the ribosome would fall off the mRNA at that point.

Kan had proven a very important point. Thalassemia could be due either to total absence of mRNA as in a gene deletion or to a severe dysfunction of mRNA as in this case. Just as sickle cell anemia is a disease brought about by a single base change in a three-base codon, so do some forms of thalassemia occur by a similar mechanism.

The stop or termination codon story did not end with the Chinese gentleman from San Francisco. Kan later found another example of a stop codon, this time at codon position 39 also in exon 1. This defect proved to represent the overwhelming majority of the thalassemia mutations found on the island of Sardinia and became a prime target of prenatal diagnosis by molecular methods. In fact, this particular defect is found in almost a fifth of the individual beta thalassemia chromosomes of Mediterranean origin.

Determination of many of the remaining point mutations that cause beta zero or beta plus thalassemia required the isolation and cloning of the beta globin genes of individual patients and careful sequencing of their bases to find a mutation that would explain the findings. Though several laboratories set about to provide such data, this was to become the giant contribution of our laboratory by Orkin, who collaborated with Haig Kazazian, a geneticist from Johns Hopkins. Kazazian was skilled at determining the restriction enzyme sites of different chromosomes 11. Their collaborative efforts were important because Orkin did not want to waste time cloning and sequencing the same gene over and over again. By choosing thalassemic genes that originated on different chromosomes 11, Orkin could reserve his efforts for genes that were likely to bear mutations that had not yet been described.

Through this collaboration, Orkin and Kazazian found that they could detect six broad subtypes of mutations in Mediterranean thalassemic genes that affect different parts of the beta gene in different ways. There were (1) promoter defects in the gene itself that reduced transcription, and therefore production of beta mRNA, to a crawl; (2) nonsense mutations that totally arrest mRNA translation on the ribosomes; (3) mutations in introns that slowed or totally arrested splicing and thereby inhibited mature mRNA production from immature mRNA; (4) insertions of un-wanted bases that cause stop codons downstream of the mutation itself; and (5) deletions of required bases that do the same thing. Finally, they detected (6) a mutation far down the gene that causes instability of mature beta mRNA. Of these six subtypes, numbers 1, 3, and 6 were apt to cause beta plus thalassemia. They were usually associated with some production of normal beta mRNA and beta globin. The others were beta zero mutations. They would not permit the translation of any beta mRNA to beta globin (figure 12).

The monumental effort of Orkin and Kazazian was published in 1982. Other laboratories also jumped into the fray, and by 1987

Sites of Beta Thalassemia Point Mutations

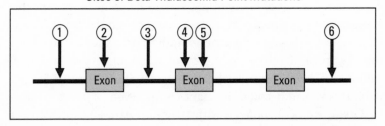

Figure 12 A point mutation in the promoter (1) reduces but usually does not stop the production of beta chain; the disease that results is called beta plus thalassemia. A nonsense mutation (2) is caused by a nu-cleotide substitution in an exon which produces a "stop" codon at the site of the mutation; stop codons result in beta zero thalassemia, where no beta chain is produced. An intron mutation (3) reduces splicing and usually results in beta plus thalassemia. A nucleotide insertion (4) or dele-tion (5) in an exon can produce a stop codon further downstream. A point mutation in the terminal end of mRNA (6) can cause instability in the molecule and lead to beta plus thalassemia.

over thirty different point mutations of the beta gene that cause thalassemia had been clearly identified. They were all variations of the six original subtypes that had been defined in 1982. By 1992 the number of different point mutations had risen to more than one hundred, all of which still represented different examples of the original six.

WHILE these studies of the mutations in the beta gene were in progress, Kazazian, Orkin, and I set about to define Dayem's particular mutation. The results were very interesting and unexpected. We knew that Dayem had beta plus thalassemia because when we first saw him he did have detectable adult hemoglobin. But because his anemia was so very severe, we thought he would have at least one beta zero gene and another beta plus. In fact, when we analyzed both of his beta clusters, we found that one of them had a subtype 3 or intron mutation in the beta gene that is detected very commonly in the Mediterranean and in the Near East. The mutation severely inhibits splicing but does not abolish it. It is a beta plus mutation. In Dayem's other beta cluster we expected a mutation that would cause beta zero thalassemia, but instead the mutation proved to be another splicing defect, a heretofore undescribed substitution that we thought should have been mild. The combination of his two splicing defects should have left him with the relatively moderate disease that Fanconi had hoped for when he first saw Dayem. Yet he had very severe anemia and terrible bone disease when I first saw him. We do not know exactly why, but the experience emphasizes the well-known fact that the clinical severity of a genetic defect does not necessarily correlate perfectly with the molecular abnormality in the gene. Other unknown factors unique to an individual influence the manifestations of the disease.

By the time we set about defining the molecular basis of Dayem's particular thalassemic defects, a remarkable advance in technology had completely changed our approach to the problem. Stuart Orkin's method of gene cloning by using plasmids had been replaced by an invention called the *polymerase chain reaction,* or

PCR. This new method was invented in 1983 by Kary Mullis, a chemist at the Cetus Corporation, a biotechnical company in California. Mullis's idea was really very simple, but most creative ideas seem simple and obvious in hindsight. It took four more years to get the kinks out of it and make it available for general use. The principle of PCR is based on the fact that certain bacteria produce enzymes that faithfully copy DNA into complementary strands. The enzymes help bacteria to reproduce themselves rapidly. By adding such an enzyme to a gene or a piece of a gene, the enzyme behaves like certain kinds of computer printers. It runs back and forth copying the last strand of DNA that it made until the operator tells it to stop. Millions of copies can be made in this fashion.

The PCR method is enormously powerful. The initial sample of DNA can be extremely small and even in poor condition. Indeed, a specific DNA sequence can be amplified from tiny samples of DNA that have been around for centuries. When we wanted to know the base sequence of Dayem's beta gene, we just amplified it up with PCR and put it through a DNA base-sequencing procedure. There was very little labor involved—almost none compared to the old methods of cloning. Cetus obtained a lucrative patent on the process, and Mullis collected a Nobel Prize for it in 1993. It is a superb invention.

One of the most important applications of PCR has been in prenatal diagnosis. If a small sample of fetal DNA can be obtained either by amniocentesis or by biopsy of the fetal portion of the placenta through the cervix, the beta gene can be amplified in any desired part, and the sequence can be determined by various direct or indirect means. If one has reliable information about the genes of the heterozygous parents, one can rather easily determine by PCR whether the fetus has inherited one, none, or both of the parents' thalassemic beta genes.

Prenatal diagnosis by these new methods has its potential sources of confusion. It is important to be certain that the amplified DNA is actually that of the fetus and not of the mother and that the putative father is the actual father. The careful laboratories that specialize in these procedures are familiar with the pitfalls. The advent of PCR has virtually abolished the need for fetal blood sampling; and in the Mediterranean countries at least, new births of thalassemic babies are continuing to decline with gratifying speed. This is now a disease that can be almost entirely prevented if screening programs and competent laboratories are established where the gene frequency is high. That has happened in Sardinia and in Greece, and those of us who had a hand in the development of these programs are very proud of the outcome.

Accurate diagnosis of the specific mutations that cause the alpha thalassemia syndromes has also developed rapidly during the past decade. The majority of these are deletions large enough to be detected by standard Southern blot analysis. Though deletional events cause most of the alpha thalassemia that is observed, particularly in the Far East, there are examples of much smaller point mutations that eradicate or markedly reduce alpha chain production. They can be detected by PCR amplification of DNA and direct or indirect sequencing of the suspected regions.

THOMAS COOLEY described thalassemia nearly seventy years ago. We began to understand its basic pathophysiology about thirty-five years ago. Twenty-five years ago we started to analyze the disease with the molecular tools that were then available to us. Fifteen years ago, we began to study the disease with ultra-modern molecular techniques that kept advancing until we can now define the precise lesion in nearly every patient we see. We can detect this disease in a very young fetus in almost every circumstance by using prenatal diagnosis, and we can offer the mother the option of selective abortion to prevent the birth of a severely ill baby.

But equally important, we have been able to transfer the knowledge that we have gained to the study of other genetic diseases and the mechanisms of normal and abnormal growth. All this has come about because patients like Dayem have given their time and their blood samples with the hope that we will find a way to help them live better lives while we advance our basic knowledge. In many ways we have earned their trust and confidence, but none of us is satisfied that our debt to them has been paid. Most of them still await a safe and simple way to be relieved of the burden of trans-fusion and chelation.

In recent years I find myself worrying about the future of the research that is so vital to the long-range survival of these patients. In our nation's understandable rush to lower the cost of medical care and to rationalize health care delivery, we may soon run the risk of crippling the small but critical academic component of health care that offers them hope of a future.

The changes in our health care system that will be necessary to free Americans from the fear of medical bankruptcy are not trivial; they will demand sacrifices from everyone, including academic physicians. Those of us in major research institutions know per-haps better than the politicians that the staggering growth of the medical establishment in the last four decades has created a vora-cious monster. When I began my internship in 1956, there were four medical schools in New England. Now there are nine medical schools and their affiliated teaching hospitals, all of which require continuous taxpayer support, insurance payments, and tuition fees to stay alive. Each of these academic institutions, in turn, produces specialists, most of whom practice privately and drive up the cost of medical care, often unnecessarily. In the near future, if our society is to provide quality health care to all Americans, everyone will have to rely much less on expensive specialists. Very careful, selective pruning of specialty practices and training programs will benefit the entire system, but short-sighted, harsh cuts will seri-ously inhibit the research productivity of the academic institutions responsible for the containment and cure of diseases in the future—some of which, like AIDS, may be unprecedented and may quickly assume epidemic proportions.

That opinion will be construed by some as the alarmist rhetoric of an unreconstructed elitist. But I'm certain that medical progress will be encumbered if we restrict research at the few institutions that have the critical mass necessary to push through biological barriers. The control of cancer and infectious diseases, the amelio-ration of inherited diseases, and the prevention of congenital de-velopmental disorders require a mastery of human genetics that is likely to be attained only in major medical centers where a highly trained corps of clinical investigators and basic researchers are supported by sufficient funds.

There are fewer than fifty such centers in the United States. In our zeal to reorganize the American medical system, we must not fail to sustain the fighting force of these institutions for the sake of the thousands of patients who, like Dayem, are waiting for a cure.

From Drugs
to Gene Therapy

AS THE 1980s UNFOLDED, a profound contrast in morale between our research laboratories and our thalassemia clinic became apparent. The laboratories were brimming with optimism. The application of molecular genetics to prenatal diagnosis had been a resounding success; new cases of thalassemia were disappearing in Greece, Sardinia, and Cyprus, proving that prenatal testing and selective abortion of severely affected fetuses could eliminate the disease. Thalassemia genes were being cloned and sequenced one after another. We were beginning to learn much more about how hemoglobin genes are turned on and off and how the red cells switch from fetal hemoglobin to adult hemoglobin production just before birth. We could actually grow large colonies of red cells in the laboratory by bathing a single bone marrow cell of a special type in certain growth factors within a culture plate. New biotechnology companies were using genetic methods to mass produce these growth factors and make them available to clinicians. We were learning to manipulate retroviruses and to insert normal hemoglobin genes into them. We hoped to coax the altered viruses to infect thalassemic bone marrow cells, where they might turn on the hemoglobin genes that they carry and thereby correct the disease. There was a future in the laboratory, and that future was almost palpable.

Meanwhile, Dayem and the other patients in our thalassemia clinic faced the same drudgery of transfusion every three weeks and the regular discomfort of daily subcutaneous Desferal. Though our excellent nurses, social workers, and blood bank technicians provided support for patients and their families and dealt with their daily problems, the older patients saw their lives as meager, unchanging, and depressing. The mood in the clinic became particularly terrible when one of the young adult patients developed heart failure. We needed new concepts of treatment, and we needed them immediately.

Complicating our search for new approaches was the financial burden borne by most of the families. Patients with thalassemia must receive red blood cell transfusions every three to four weeks and nightly infusions of one to two grams of Desferal. The cost of the blood and Desferal alone was close to $30,000 per year, to say nothing of the clinic nurses, social workers, and physicians who were needed to carefully evaluate the patients and detect physical or emotional complications before they became catastrophes.

Dayem's family had the resources to pay for his treatment without hardship, but most of the families were of modest means. Stephen D. was a sheet-metal worker, and John C. was a plumber. Among the young adults, Susan, a high school student, was the daughter of a state university administrator, and Jackie's father was in middle management; Olga was a medical secretary; Fatima was a college student whose father practiced public service law.

Families like these can be cruelly abused by the porous American health care system. They are often cut off from coverage by insurance carriers that seek to avoid such expensive responsibilities, leaving families pauperized by medical debt and their hospitals and doctors to provide free care. Small wonder that the parents of most American children with thalassemia appear careworn and sometimes exhausted. Not only is the disease incurable in the standard sense, it is terribly time-consuming and stressful to manage and can bankrupt a family. Were it not for a relatively small federal grant-in-aid to states that supports some of the treatment of children with crippling diseases, and the devotion of a few hospitals and physicians in New York, Pennsylvania, California, and New England where most of the patients reside, the pressure on most parents would be too great to bear.

In settings such as these, associations of parents and patients are formed to provide mutual support, share ideas and experiences with similarly afflicted families, raise money for research through private donations, and lobby legislatures for funds. The American Heart Association and the American Cancer Society are perhaps the most visible of these organizations. The Cooley's Anemia Foundation, by contrast, is a small group begun in New York by Italian-Americans who hope for substantial progress in thalassemia research before their own children succumb. Their lobbying efforts have been successful. They have been able to persuade Congress to allocate money for thalassemia research and treatment by inserting specific language into the bills that actually fund the various institutes of the National Institutes of Health. Such a result is not easily achieved. It requires ceaseless attention to key representatives and often financial support of their election expenses. The activity provides an opportunity for society members to join together and channel their grief and worry into something practical and realizable. I've come to admire them, even though they can be vociferous in their demands and occasionally unrealistic in their expectations.

In response to the needs of our patients and their families and to our own frustration, we searched desperately for new treatment ideas, particularly for the older patients like Dayem. We focused our efforts on four promising areas: *bone marrow transplantation* (described earlier), an approach that would apply only to the relatively few patients who might have compatible donors; the development of an *orally active iron chelator* (examples of which have already been described); the stimulation of *fetal hemoglobin synthesis* to replace deficient production of the beta chains of adult hemoglobin; and the transfer of normal functioning globin genes into the patients' bone marrow cells (so-called *gene transfer therapy*).

Treatment of thalassemia by stimulation of fetal hemoglobin production is based on the fact that thalassemia is a disorder of unbalanced hemoglobin synthesis. In beta thalassemia, the primary problem is a deficiency of beta globin chains, and therefore inadequate formation of adult hemoglobin, in the red cell. A second and very serious problem is the accumulation of unmatched alpha chains that damage the red cell membrane and cause rapid destruction of the developing red cell within the bone marrow. As we saw in the cases of Mr. Zhanghi, Stephen, and John, the globin chain imbalance can be less damaging if the defect in beta chain production is relatively mild or if the production of the gamma chains of fetal hemoglobin is somehow accelerated. At this time, we cannot modify beta chain production in thalassemia. That would require transfer of a functioning globin gene into a patient's stem cells, a technology that is not yet ready for clinical trials. In contrast, we *can* modify gamma chain production through drug therapy, and have been doing so for years. That story is linked to our knowledge of the fetal switch.

THE FAILURE of thalassemia beta genes to switch on just before birth, as they are supposed to do, is not obvious in newborns because the infants' red cells are still filled with fetal hemoglobin, the synthesis of which predominates during intra-uterine life (see figure 6 on page 32). As gamma chain synthesis switches off after birth, the deficiency of beta chain production and the accumulation of unmatched alpha chains steadily worsens until anemia is apparent. But in some unusual cases, patients maintain high levels of fetal hemoglobin production long after birth. This suggests that the severity of symptoms could be lessened, and perhaps even eliminated, if gamma chain production could somehow be made to persist instead of switching off.

For that reason a tremendous amount of research has been focused on (1) the precise molecular mechanism of the fetal switch that turns off fetal hemoglobin production in normal people, (2) those conditions under which fetal hemoglobin production naturally increases in some thalassemic patients, and (3) drugs that might stimulate fetal hemoglobin production in the other cases of thalassemia. As a result of all of this effort, we now know much more about the switching mechanism. We lack some very important details and it is very complex, but the general outline of the system is becoming clear.

An immature bone marrow cell, called a stem cell, becomes a committed producer of red cells when certain nuclear proteins—

called *transcription factors*—attach themselves to specific short stretches or domains of DNA. One important class of transcription factors are *enhancer-binding proteins*. When enhancer-binding proteins adhere to enhancer domains in the DNA, they switch the globin genes on and off at the right time and in the right order. The "on switch" is further governed by other transcription factors that bind to specific short stretches or domains of DNA called *promoters*, which are just upstream of the globin genes and initiate transcription. For many genes, other nuclear proteins *repress* transcription; when they bind to specific stretches of DNA bases, transcription ceases. The short stretches of DNA to which nuclear transcription factors such as enhancers, promoters, and repressors bind are not found in exons, though enhancer-binding domains may be located in introns. Most enhancer-binding domains are upstream of the structural gene. Some are very far upstream.

In the beta globin cluster of genes on chromosome 11 (see figure 11 on page 177), the first gene to be tapped by nuclear proteins is the epsilon gene, which provides the beta-like half of the hemoglobin molecules in the red cells of the embryo. Very soon the epsilon gene is switched off, and the gamma gene of fetal hemoglobin is switched on. Finally, enhancers switch on the beta gene, and switch off the gamma. In effect, the individual members of this group of beta globin genes, lined up from left to right, turn on and off one after another during fetal development because they are tapped by enhancers to start and finish their expression at certain times in a sequence, like red, yellow, and green traffic lights.

Every two years a small group of experts on hemoglobin gathers for three days to discuss how this fetal switch works. The "switch meeting" is a quasi-sacred event for those who have contemplated this problem for decades. Inevitably, at some point during those three days the conversation turns to a remarkable phenomenon that hematologists have known about for years: Whenever humans or primates have a sudden burst of increased red cell production, such as after a substantial hemorrhage or during the recovery phase of a bone marrow transplant, gamma chain production dramatically reactivates. Fetal hemoglobin may rise to as high as 10 percent of the total hemoglobin; and more than 50 percent of the cells will have detectable fetal hemoglobin. Normally, the level of fetal hemoglobin in adult blood is less than one percent; and no more than 10 or 15 percent of the circulating red cells have any detectable fetal hemoglobin at all.

Furthermore, if bone marrow cells taken from a normal adult who has a very low circulating level of fetal hemoglobin are cultured in a dish with appropriate growth factors, colonies of red cells will be produced that express much higher levels of fetal hemoglobin than adults ordinarily do. This laboratory experiment further substantiates the conclusion drawn from observing living patients: that accelerated red cell production causes a rise in fetal hemoglobin synthesis. But how does the acceleration of red cell production stimulate the gamma genes? We still don't have the answer.

A few years ago at one of those biennial meetings, members of Arthur Nienhuis's laboratory at the National Institutes of Health announced the results of a remarkable piece of clinical investigation using an anticancer drug called 5-aza-cytidine. Investigators at a Veterans Administration hospital in Chicago had already shown that the drug stimulates fetal hemoglobin production in baboons. With some courage, I thought, Nienhuis and his group (in association with other colleagues at Johns Hopkins) administered 5-aza-cytidine to a few patients with thalassemia and sickle cell anemia. A definite increase in gamma chain production was observed in some! That was big news. No one had previously used a drug to stimulate gamma chain production in patients with disorders of hemoglobin. Our world of experimental hematologists was electrified by these results.

When the results of the experiments were published in the prestigious *New England Journal of Medicine,* Edward Benz, then at Yale, wrote a stirring editorial in which he announced that molecular biology had been brought to the bedside. The fact that DNA could be fooled into incorporating a drug that in turn would stimulate fetal hemoglobin production meant that a new era of molecular therapy was before us.

I agreed that the experiment was very important, but I did not agree with that interpretation. The effectiveness of this drug as an anticancer agent was due to its ability to stop cells from dividing.

(What all cancers have in common is the uncontrolled division and multiplication of cells.) When this drug is administered to cultured cell lines that are rapidly dividing in a flask in the laboratory, for example, it arrests cell division and the cells die. The reasons for this effect are somewhat complicated but they all stem from the fact that cells confuse 5-aza-cytidine for its parent compound, normal cytidine, and incorporate it into their DNA. It seemed to me that *any* drug that inhibits red-cell division—by any means— would have the same effect of stimulating fetal hemoglobin production, whether it is incorporated into DNA or not.

Furthermore, I was concerned about the future of 5-aza-cytidine in therapy. That drug has some very serious side effects and had been virtually removed from the anticancer drug list for that reason. I did not think that we would ever be able to justify its use in a nonmalignant condition, though thalassemia is a wretched illness and risks are required in a desperate circumstance.

On the other hand, I thought that the general approach was intriguing. If we treated patients intermittently with a drug that would temporarily inhibit the division of red cell precursors in the marrow, would red cell production not only recover but actually speed up when the drug was stopped? And would this off-on effect stimulate them to turn on their gamma genes and keep them on long enough to build up fetal hemoglobin in many of the newly formed red cells? If so, would those cells rich in fetal hemoglobin persist in the blood? To borrow a phrase from David Weatherall, I decided to "have a go at it," and I chose hydroxyurea as the ideal drug.

Hydroxyurea is a very simple compound. It is a small molecule that is actually a minor modification of urea, the compound that is excreted in the urine carrying the body's excess nitrogen. Hydroxyurea may have occurred to me because its mode of action as an antileukemia drug is to bind iron very tightly and in so doing inhibit production of an iron-dependent enzyme, without which cells cannot divide. Fortunately for patients, hydroxyurea has a rapid and reversible effect on cells. It is not incorporated into DNA. Its influence disappears quickly unless the dose is repeatedly renewed. Hence it is a relatively safe drug, but one that is not widely used because its range of effectiveness is limited. It works quite well in a few kinds of leukemia, but poorly in most.

Given the fact that, at the very least, hydroxyurea is a considerably less toxic way than 5-aza-cytidine to inhibit cell division, I decided to join forces with Norman Letvin, chief of immunology at the New England Primate Center, and Peter Beardsley and David Linch in my laboratory to organize a series of experiments with the drug using crab-eating monkeys (macaca fascicularis) as models. Beardsley is now chief of pediatric hematology at Yale, and Linch is chief at University College Hospital in London. The monkeys were first bled until they were anemic like our patients. Then they were given hydroxyurea at different doses, which suddenly arrested red cell production. When the hydroxyurea was withdrawn, the results were striking. The monkeys made vast amounts of fetal hemoglobin. After weeks of this off-on treatment, nearly every one of their red cells contained fetal hemoglobin. Now we had proven that a drug that inhibits cell division *without being incorporated into DNA* could stimulate fetal hemoglobin synthesis in animals with anemia and accelerated red cell production. We next had to find out whether the drug would work in humans.

To make that step, we had to ask ourselves about the proper choice of patients. In my heart, I did not really think that the approach would be helpful in thalassemia. The required increase in fetal hemoglobin would be considerably higher than anything we could responsibly hope to achieve by manipulating the fetal switch in this way. To treat thalassemia, the level of hemoglobin in the blood has to be kept high enough to shut off the red cell assembly lines in the bone marrow. Otherwise, the bone marrow spaces continue to enlarge in order to produce more and more of their defective red cells, and the bones become weaker and weaker. To lower the transfusion requirement in thalassemia would demand a very large positive stimulation of gamma chain production, one that would virtually fill the cell with gamma chains that could pair with the excess alpha chains. Even a doubling or tripling of gamma chain production would not be sufficient in most cases. We would need at least a five-fold increase to achieve a therapeutic effect.

Sickle cell anemia was another matter, and more promising. Fetal hemoglobin has a curious effect on the red cells of patients with sickle cell anemia. A relatively small amount of fetal hemoglobin actually inhibits sickle hemoglobin from assuming a sickle shape. If we could achieve a two- to three-fold increase in fetal hemoglobin in the majority of red cells in patients with sickle cell anemia, we might expect symptoms to decrease markedly.

To carry out the first study of hydroxyurea in sickle cell disease, I turned to Dr. Orah Platt, then a member of our clinic and laboratory who had become our resident expert in sickle cell anemia. Platt is now the Director of Clinical Laboratories at Children's Hospital. She conducted an exciting study which established that hydroxyurea would indeed stimulate fetal hemoglobin in that disease and seemed to improve the anemia as well. Her findings were confirmed and considerably extended by colleagues at Johns Hopkins, who have recently mounted a national clinical trial to determine whether hydroxyurea can reduce the incidence of painful episodes and the other miserable manifestations of sickle cell disease. So far, that trial, as well as a smaller study by French physicians, is very encouraging. In about half the patients, the incidence of painful crisis is greatly decreased.

At this writing, we don't know exactly how useful or toxic hydroxyurea will prove to be in sickle cell disease, and we doubt that it will be helpful at all in thalassemia. But at least we established a very important principle: that drugs can be used to manipulate the human fetal switch. That discovery has stimulated further experiments, this time with butyric acid, a completely natural fatty compound in the body that makes tennis shoes smelly in the summer.

The notion that butyric acid might be useful in thalassemia arose from simple observations of the offspring of mothers with diabetes. Infants born to diabetic mothers are usually very large because a high level of blood sugar in the mother stimulates the fetus's pancreas to release excessive amounts of insulin. Insulin promotes fat accumulation when there is an adequate source of calories. Therefore, the babies of diabetic mothers are very fat. But these babies also have another peculiarity: They have high circulating levels of butyric acid and elevated fetal hemoglobin levels for their gestational age.

The high fetal hemoglobin in such infants made Susan Perrine and Douglas Faller in our division of hematology and oncology very curious about its cause. Susan came by her curiosity quite honestly because her father is Dr. Richard Perrine, who was for many years a physician in the ARAMCO oil fields in Dhahran, a town in the oil-producing Eastern Province of Saudi Arabia. During his long tenure with ARAMCO, Richard Perrine made a startling observation. Working in the blistering and desiccating heat of the oil fields were men with sickle cell anemia! Indeed, the indigenous Arab population is loaded with sickle cell disease, alpha thalassemia, and some beta thalassemia, all signs of a population in which malaria had been rampant.

The Persian Gulf littoral of the Eastern Province is a huge swampy oasis in which the anopheles mosquito reigned supreme. The bedouins knew better than to sleep there. They tried to pitch their tents in the desert right behind the oasis so they could be free of the insects. Nonetheless, the anopheles mosquito picked them off, killing with particular frequency those with normal hemoglobin genes and leaving behind many carriers of sickle cell anemia and thalassemia whose genetic mutations offered some protection against malaria. For that reason, the frequency of hemoglobin mutations in the present generation is very high.

What was fascinating to Perrine was the fact that men with sickle cell anemia could work so well in the dry heat of the desert. If there is one massive danger to patients with sickle cell anemia, it is the combination of dehydration and heat. Even patients with mere sickle cell trait (those with only one sickle beta gene) can be seriously injured by extremes of heat and dehydration. The United States Air Force proved that point dramatically one sad day when they flew some new recruits to a base in the high elevations of Colorado in particularly hot, dry weather. They then ordered a vigorous exercise drill. When several of the black recruits collapsed, they called a halt, but not before two deaths occurred. Those men had sickle cell trait. The combination of heat, severe dehydration, and the slight anoxia of altitude had caused their red cells to sickle because the rate and extent of sickling is an inverse function of oxygen pressure and a direct function of the concentration of sickle hemoglobin and temperature.

When Richard Perrine saw bedouins with two sickle beta genes working under conditions that should have killed them, he rubbed his eyes with disbelief and then set about to find out why they survived. To his amazement, he found that those particular workers had extraordinarily high levels of fetal hemoglobin. The average level of fetal hemoglobin in an American black with sickle cell anemia is about 8 percent of the total hemoglobin; the average in Perrine's Saudis was above 20 percent!

For many years, American scientists have been searching for a drug that can be orally absorbed, enter red cells, and inhibit the ability of sickle hemoglobin to assume the rod-like shape that it readily assumes when oxygen is low, hemoglobin concentration is high, and temperature is elevated. The best antisickling agent that has ever been found is fetal hemoglobin. A red cell may be nearly full of sickle hemoglobin, but if there is at least 15 percent of fetal hemoglobin accompanying the sickle hemoglobin in the cell, the sickle hemoglobin will tend to remain in a globular form, and the red cell will retain its flexible shape. Therefore, fetal hemoglobin is an antisickling agent par excellence, and these Eastern Oasis Saudis were loaded with it. They could work in those terrible conditions, and many did quite well, though some of the workers did get ill from time to time.

I became very interested in this remarkable group of Saudis, and so did my friend David Weatherall. Together we decided on an approach to learn more about the fetal switch by studying them and their families very carefully. We enlisted the excellent skills of Dr. Barbara Miller, who worked in my laboratory at the time and is now Professor of Pediatrics at Pennsylvania State University in Hershey. With the help of colleagues from the ARAMCO Hospital in Dhahran, Barbara obtained blood samples from families in the Dhahran community, some of whom had sickle cell anemia, some sickle trait, and others with entirely normal levels of fetal and adult hemoglobin.

The blood samples were shipped by air to my laboratory in Boston, where Barbara isolated from each of them the rare population of cells that can, with certain growth factors, multiply into colonies of red cells. These are actually bone marrow cells, very few of which normally escape from the marrow and circulate in the blood. When Barbara measured the amounts of fetal and adult hemoglobin in the colonies, she found extraordinarily high levels of fetal hemoglobin in the red cell colonies derived from many members of the Eastern Oasis families, even those who did not have sickle trait. Their tendency to make high levels of fetal hemoglobin proved to be due to a subtle but favorable second hemoglobin gene mutation, this one in the promoter of one of their gamma genes.

As already mentioned, promoters are short sequences of bases found at the beginning of many genes, from bacteria to humans, which, in concert with enhancers, regulate transcription. This particular promoter mutation is frequently found in the Oasis, in the Orissa province of India, and in regions of Africa as well. Wherever it exists, fetal hemoglobin production is high; and when it is inherited in conjunction with sickle cell anemia, the sickle disease is mild because fetal hemoglobin is increased in the red cell. This combination of mutations, which protects from both malaria and sickle cell symptoms, was highly favored by natural selection in this hot, dry, mosquito-infested part of the world.

The story of those Saudi oil workers with sickle cell anemia had always fascinated Susan Perrine; she had heard her father talk about them endlessly. She began to wonder whether drugs other than hydroxyurea might be broadly effective in stimulating fetal hemoglobin synthesis in patients with sickle cell anemia or thalassemia, whether or not they had inherited the Eastern Oasis promoter mutation. That was why she decided to examine the infants of diabetic mothers more carefully. "What substance," she asked (somewhat naively, I thought), "could be circulating in those mothers that would stimulate gamma chain production?"

DREADING an endless search for an evanescent compound, I advised Susan to stay away from the problem and do more conservative experiments that would produce a definitive answer quickly.

I've been in the business of training young physician-scientists for more than thirty years. It's a satisfying task, but it can be very difficult. Young physicians have a hard road before them if they are to become successful in research. First of all, they are much older than most non-MD-holding graduate students when they begin work in the laboratory. After four years of college, four years of medical school, and four more years of internship, residency, and clinical fellowship training, they are often above the age of thirty when they begin to learn something about molecular research. That's the age when mathematicians are thinking about retirement!

At my age, academic physicians often look back at a previous era with a fondness for privation that is probably fostered by geriatric amnesia. When I get into a discussion with a nascent physician-scientist like Susan Perrine, my opinion about her plans is either consciously or unconsciously influenced by my own experience. It is important, however, to understand that one must view past experience in the context of the period in which the experience was gained. Young people are often given poor advice by those who romanticize their earlier years.

My era of training was in the 1950s when the science of clinical medicine was much simpler than today. It was relatively easy to learn the high clinical technology of that period because there wasn't very much of it. Basic science was also much simpler before the application of molecular genetics in the biomedical sciences. One could be a pretty good clinical scientist and develop a national reputation by applying the biochemistry of the 1950s and 1960s to a deeper understanding of patients with unexplained diseases. These patients had already been categorized and catalogued by the then clinical greats such as Louis K. Diamond at Children's Hospital in Boston or Sir John Dacie at the Hammersmith Hospital in London. To become recognized as a future leader, one had to be in a hospital to which interesting patients were referred, have excellent clinical skills in distinguishing one kind of patient problem from another, and have enough biochemical training to measure proteins and various salts and metabolites with techniques that would now be considered primitive in modern clinical laboratories.

In fact, a good many of us were simply scratching the surface of science. We were more akin to strip miners than to deep-shaft miners. Because our basic scientific training was rather skimpy, we tended to focus on patients from whom we could get rapid answers, rather than digging deeply into a scientific question that might require more technical knowledge and skill than we could hope to acquire in a reasonable period of time. Time was important. We were long in the tooth as scientists go. We had to choose projects that would work after an acceptable length of effort. Otherwise, even in that era of less intense grant competition, we would be left behind academically and financially. Finances were a particular problem. We received so little salary that we could not support a family without the assistance of our parents or our spouses. With some help, however, our finances were just bearable because we had paid relatively little for our college and medical school educations.

Despite the tendency of members of my age group to look back on their own struggles as the hardest of times, the difficulties young clinical scientists face today are much greater. Our trainees are paid far better than we were, but their housing costs are comparatively horrendous, and their educational debts are horrifying. It is not unusual to meet a first-year fellow in the laboratory who is supporting a wife and a couple of young kids, has taken on a mortgage debt exceeding $100,000, and at the same time is trying to pay back an educational loan of that much or more. These folks are forced to moonlight in community hospital emergency rooms to keep their monthly housing payments going.

Furthermore, as scientists they have a lot of catching up to do. Their medical school educations have not provided them with the depth of scientific training that they need to compete in laboratory research unless they have completed M.D.-Ph.D. programs. These double-degree programs require even more time and are themselves only variably successful, but at least they are federally funded and students who emerge from them are free of medical school tuition debt. Even if today's students do learn some useful science in medical school, they are faced with three to four years of clinical training with increasingly complex technology. Once they get all that behind them, they must then find a way to become very good at modern molecular biology. The technical skills required, and the knowledge underlying them, cannot be mastered quickly.

Finally, they face a competition for research grants that has become awesome. The research enterprise has outstripped its resources, and young people in excellent institutions are having a desperate time getting funded. The number of physician-scientists who are successful in that fierce competition is declining rapidly.

Small wonder that I was very cautious with Susan Perrine when she told me that she wanted to search for some unnamed compound in the blood of infants of diabetic mothers that might stimulate fetal hemoglobin production. I listened a bit more carefully, however, when she and Doug Faller, who was then one of our assistant professors and is now the Director of the Boston University Cancer Center, suggested that the search might be rapid if the compound was, as they already guessed, butyric acid. They decided on butyric acid because it is elevated in the blood of infants of diabetic mothers and because it is known to bind to DNA.

To examine the effects of butyric acid on gamma chain synthesis, Susan Perrine collaborated with Barbara Miller to study its influence on fetal hemoglobin synthesis in the red cell colonies that Barbara produced in the laboratory. To their delight, there was a substantial increase in gamma chain synthesis and fetal hemoglobin accumulation in those colonies when butyric acid was added to the culture system.

Susan subsequently took a position at the Oakland Children's Hospital and shortly thereafter did a remarkable experiment with a group of physiologists at the University of California at San Francisco. The physiologists were interested in the development of the sheep fetus and could make a very useful maternal-fetal sheep model by dexterously placing and maintaining small plastic tubes in the blood vessels of the sheep fetus during the last half of pregnancy. This set-up permitted Susan to infuse the fetus with butyric acid and measure the fetal hemoglobin produced by the sheep fetus.

Normally, the sheep fetus turns off its production of fetal hemoglobin shortly before birth, and the total circulating fetal hemoglobin progressively declines after birth. In that limited sense sheep are very much like humans. To everyone's amazement except Susan's (who confidently expected it), some of the sheep who received butyric acid never turned off their fetal hemoglobin production at all. Somehow, the butyric acid had blocked the fetal switch!

When I heard about that result, I was very impressed. So were all the fetal hemoglobin aficionados who attend the biennial switch meeting. Susan's work was the subject of intense discussion. Before long, she and Barbara began to examine sickle cell anemia and thalassemia red cell colonies in the laboratory and found that these red cells contained considerably more fetal hemoglobin when they were incubated in the presence of butyric acid.

All of these results persuaded the United States Food and Drug Administration to encourage Susan and Doug Faller to search for compounds related to butyric acid that might be just as active or even more active but would circulate in the plasma for a longer period and be less smelly. That work is now in progress, and a few patients have actually been treated with butyric acid itself. The results in one patient with thalassemia intermedia are quite impressive. She received a prolonged treatment with the compound and experienced a rapid rise in fetal hemoglobin and a decrease in the rate at which she destroyed red cells in the marrow.

It is much too soon to know whether butyric acid will offer a therapeutic advantage to many patients with thalassemia. In fact, a recently performed evaluation of the drug by Nancy Olivieri in Toronto suggests that it will have very limited—if any—utility. Furthermore, a drug such as butyric acid is very nonspecific. It is likely to have wide and possibly toxic influences on gene expression in unwanted places. We really don't want some of our genes to be talking all the time. But butyric acid can on occasion influence gamma gene expression; and on the rare occasions when it does work, it is certainly superior to hydroxyurea, at least in thalassemia.

Despite our enthusiasm for the new drug treatments of either sickle cell disease or thalassemia, including orally active iron chelators, hydroxyurea, and butyric acid, they all represent halfway measures that require continuous treatment, monitoring of toxicity, and substantial if not prohibitive cost. What is needed is a safe and sure cure that would end the disease in a given individual and permit most of our attention to focus on the prevention of new cases.

BONE MARROW transplantation from a compatible donor is just such an approach, but it is very limited in scope because it can only be performed in the minority of patients who have compatible donors. And even in those cases many patients fail, largely because of recurrence of thalassemia, infection, or graft-versus-host disease. Bone marrow transplants are, however, a form of gene therapy that works. We don't replace one gene when we do a bone marrow transplant, however; we replace an entire group of cells—all the cells of the marrow, with all of their genes. That is unfortunate, because thalassemia is a disease that is expressed only in red cells. The fact that a patient's globin genes are abnormal makes not a whit of difference to his or her platelets, white cells, and immune cells, all of which function normally. And when we replace all of a person's blood-cell-producing machinery, we then have to deal with all of the cellular products that those transplanted bone marrow cells manufacture. Graft-versus-host disease, in which the immune cells—called lymphocytes—from the bone marrow graft attack the patient (rather than the other way around, as happens in rejection), is the worst outcome of the nonspecific nature of bone marrow transplants.

If we could select marrow cells for transplantation that give rise *only* to red cells, we could avoid graft-versus-host disease entirely because red cells have nothing to do with immunity. However, there are no primitive and continuously sustaining marrow cells that give rise solely to red cells. In order to achieve a sustained graft of marrow, we have to transplant the whole crowd. More selective engraftment may be possible in the future, but right now the only way to achieve near 100 percent engraftment and avoid graft-versus-host disease is to perform a bone marrow *autotransplant*.

Autotransplantation is now particularly well accepted in the treatment of certain kinds of childhood leukemia—malignancies in which white blood cells reproduce uncontrollably. After standard chemotherapy, some of the child's bone marrow is removed and treated with special antibodies or other drugs that are designed to remove any residual leukemia cells that might be present. The child then receives a very large dose of antileukemic drugs and sometimes irradiation, all intended to kill off the remaining leukemia cells in his body. Finally, the cleansed marrow is returned to its putatively cancer-free marrow space, where production of normal blood cells resumes. In our hands, the results of autotransplantation among leukemia patients are almost as good as the results of sibling donor transplantation; and since the transplanted tissues come from the host's own body, graft-versus-host disease is avoided.

In adults, this approach is currently being evaluated as a form of treatment for resistant tumors of the breast, lung, genito-urinary tract, and gastrointestinal tract. After the marrow is removed and stored, very large doses of chemotherapy are given to kill all of the cancer cells in the body. They usually fail to do so, but these anticancer-cell drugs are so potent that they destroy any marrow cells that remain in the body, which is why healthy marrow must be harvested and preserved before the chemotherapy begins. The marrow (in some trials experimentally cleansed of any tumor cells it might contain) is then returned to the patient. There is preliminary evidence that the method may extend the lives of certain adult patients with solid tumors, but it needs more evaluation.

These are all very interesting therapeutic ideas, but on the surface at least autotransplantation does not seem to apply to the thalassemia problem. If we destroy the patient's bone marrow with chemotherapy and then reinsert his stored marrow, we will simply recreate thalassemia, since the mutation still resides in the genes of the transplanted cells. So if autotransplantation is to be used in the treatment of thalassemia or sickle cell disease, we will have to modify the stored marrow, and the modification must involve inserting a normal beta globin gene into the tiny number of stem cells that are in the stored marrow sample. It won't do the patient any good to correct the established red cells that are in the stored sample because they have a finite life span and will eventually die. Only suitable alterations of the rare stem cells that have the mysterious capacity to both renew themselves and differentiate to all blood cells, including red cells, can provide continuous correction of thalassemia for the lifetime of the patient.

Though the concept of such a cure is exciting and challenging, many serious barriers stand in the way. In a sample of a million marrow cells, there may be one stem cell. A major problem is to find that cell. Then we have to insert a functioning beta globin gene into it, usually carried by a retrovirus. Finally, the beta globin gene has to be normally expressed when the marrow-reconstituting cell becomes an early red cell (which means that all the regulatory elements surrounding the structural gene have to be functioning properly). All of this is a very tall scientific order on which many laboratories are working, thus far without success. The very few marrow-reconstituting stem cells that can be isolated from samples do not take up retroviruses bearing beta globin genes very well; and when they do, the globin genes are poorly expressed in early red cells. But the concept is a tremendous opportunity for the new field of molecular medicine and one that fascinates many bright young minds.

I believe that gene transfer therapy will one day be useful in certain inherited diseases and that limited success might be achieved within a decade of hard work. Will thalassemia be the first to be corrected? I doubt it, but I have the pride of knowing that the problem of thalassemia stimulated the movement toward gene replacement therapy just as it began the application of molecular biology in medicine. I hope that we will be ready one day soon with this great advance. Meanwhile, transfusion, chelation, and—in a few appropriate circumstances—bone marrow transplantation remain the best approaches that we can offer our patients now.

Closing In

DAYEM SAIF is one of the most likeable patients I have ever known, despite the mask of insouciance he wears and the bad habits he adopted during his teenage years. I don't believe that he ever deliberately lied to me, and I am sure that when he returned to Washington in 1981, he believed he would keep his pledge to take the Desferal. But his lifestyle made it impossible for him to comply. The whole concept of overnight drug dosing is built on the fairly reasonable assumption that people go to bed at night and sleep. I do. Even my teenage daughters did, though I always worried about the company they might keep.

Perhaps it was the stress of being a parent of teenagers in the late 1960s and 1970s that gave me some understanding of what Dayem and his parents were going through as they tried to make him accept the cumbersome treatment. My children entered the adolescent storm at a time when every accepted social norm was being shattered. Canons of patriotism, race, class, and education that were so clear to my generation were collapsing before our eyes. As young Americans in the era of World War II, most of my generation devoutly believed in the United States as the sentinel and savior of the free world. We had stood against the most terrible tyrants in history and vanquished them. Representatives of the United States government were honored in our families. Roosevelt and Truman were nearly sanctified. Eisenhower was seen as dull but above personal criticism. John Kennedy was a thoughtful and humorous young president, whose freshness and idealism made us feel optimistic about the future. Until his assassination, all was right in our well-ordered world except the growing threat of Soviet expansion.

Then came the ugly chasms of Vietnam and the increasing awareness of widespread racism. Our children no longer believed in Sanctuary America. They came into adolescence without a social or community anchor. As they strode about in black pajama-like costumes inspired by the Viet Cong, they had to find themselves without the solidity of fixed, albeit naive, beliefs. Many were lost— never discovering a sense of self in time. I feel very fortunate that my children made it through that mine field relatively unscathed.

In the many conversations I had with Dayem, I came to understand that chronic illness played an enormous additional role in his adolescent explosion. For good reason, he lacked confidence in any future at all, and he was desperate to join a group that would accept him. His face was corrected, but his inner view of himself was of a sickly, transfusion-dependent little boy. It was obvious that he could not add to that burden by hooking himself to a pump instead of enjoying a wild night of blaring music and cannabis-inspired fantasies.

I talked for hours with Mrs. Saif about our mutual frustration. "At least," she would utter wryly, "I don't have to worry about whether he is sleeping alone at night, because he never goes to bed at all until dawn." She was correct on that point. After a night of carousing in every disco in and around Washington, he would collapse wherever he happened to be and sleep the clock around until the next night's activities began. His family tried every maneuver known to all parents in an effort to change his habits, but it was hopeless. Dayem seemed to be out on an endless spree. Threats to cut him off were useless; his illness made that impossible. So we all decided to hunker down and wait for the adolescent pestilence to drift away like a toxic cloud. Meanwhile, he continued to ignore our instructions, coming to the NIH for his blood transfusions and slinking away before the physicians there could berate him for his failure to take the Desferal.

On one of his visits to our clinic, he confessed that he had not used the Desferal pump more than a few times since he had returned to Washington. Angrily, I admitted him for another month of intravenous high-dose Desferal. I hoped to wash out as much iron as I could. Indeed, grams of iron were removed, and he began once again on the subcutaneous program, but I knew he wouldn't stay with it. Therefore, I persuaded him to remain in the hospital for yet another month that summer for extended treatment.

At that time, I began to notice some subtle changes in his attitude. True, the parade of young ladies continued, but he seemed to spend hours on the telephone talking about *deals*. This time the deals had nothing to do with entertainment, and—much to my relief—nothing to do with illegal drugs. He was actually talking via a portable phone to hospitals in the Near East and to manufacturers of hospital equipment and construction supplies in the United States. He was seeking investors for medical inventions that he had caught wind of during his long sojourns in the hospital. Dayem, the playboy, was becoming Dayem, the business-dealmaker. He was beginning to see himself as a person with a future. Perhaps, if I could take a more distant posture, he could begin to work out some sort of a life for himself that might include a certain level of compliance—enough at least to protect his heart for a few more years. On the other hand, I also knew that we would have to find a way to persuade him to take the drug on a daily basis. He still hated the subcutaneous route and complained bitterly of the pain. We needed constant intravenous access. It would soon be time for the surgeons to lend a hand.

I took the first step by asking the surgeons to fashion a connection or shunt between a large vein and a moderate-sized artery in his groin. I reasoned that the rapid blood flow through the vein would expand it and make it very easy for Dayem to insert a needle and infuse himself constantly with Desferal, using the portable pump on a 24-hour basis. I repeatedly warned him to employ scrupulously clean technique, to wash his hands, clean the skin, cover the needle, replace it daily or every other day at the most, and, above all, to do the procedure regularly because his heart demanded it.

In addition to that plan, I decided to offer him an entirely different kind of red cell transfusion program. As he turned twenty-one, the transfusion service began to transfuse him by machine. They would insert a needle into blood vessels and pump his blood into a centrifuge that would spin it and discard his old red cells—those that were about to die and deposit their iron in his body. Now depleted of their oldest members, the centrifuged red cells were then returned to a vein, accompanied by a dose of very young red cells that we had scooped from the blood of a donor. Those young red cells would live for several weeks in his body. We would repeat the procedure two months later in order to remove more red cells before they died. We called his old red cells gerocytes, and the new ones that we gave him neocytes. The procedure was called a neocyte-gerocyte exchange. I calculated that his annual transfusion-induced iron load would be reduced 25 percent by that complex procedure, and any significant reduction might help him now. It would only be useful, however, if he would cooperate and take intravenous Desferal all day and every day through the new venoarterial connection in his groin.

I was disappointed, but not surprised, when in August of 1983, a few months after his twenty-first birthday, Dayem went into severe heart failure for the first time. He awakened from a sound sleep very short of breath. He sat upright but remained symptomatic. The symptoms worsened, and he reported to the nearest emergency room, the one at Georgetown University Hospital. There the doctors were nonplussed to say the least. This young man's history and his treatment plan were so complex that very few physicians would have seen anything like him. But Georgetown University physicians knew heart failure when they saw it. They treated him vigorously and very effectively for two days and then thankfully shipped him to Boston for his seventeenth admission to Children's Hospital.

The physical examination was ominous. His skin was dark brown, his liver and heart were enlarged, his lungs had evidence of fluid in the air sacs, and the veins of his neck were distended. All of these findings were consistent with the toxicity of iron overload and its attendant heart failure. Obviously he had not used the new shunt on a regular basis. Intensive treatment with antibiotics in case of an infection and with drugs that improve cardiac function was begun, but the fundamental issue—Dayem's unwillingness or inability to infuse himself constantly with Desferal—remained the central problem.

As we were debating our next approach, another disaster struck. The shunt in his groin clotted. Probably Dayem's heart failure reduced the blood flow in the shunt to the point at which clotting was initiated, but repeated injections through it had also compromised the vessels. Now we had no convenient access to his circulation except through the smaller peripheral veins in his arms, and these had been heavily used. I felt that we were being closed in by the limits of anatomy. Veins and arteries need to be left alone. They cannot be repeatedly punctured without damage. Vital tissues cannot be loaded with iron. We were using halfway or quarterway measures to deal with a fundamental problem, and each of the incomplete measures had its own set of complications. So we were managing the complications of our treatment rather than the basic problem itself.

Somehow Dayem kept our spirits afloat. On the surface, the clotting of the shunt didn't seem to be the end of the world for him. "We'll have to do something else, Doc," he offered. But I could see a certain change in him. He would still laugh easily when I came into the room. We could still exchange our ideas about Palestinians and Israelis, and I could still yell at him about Desferal. But there was a growing and unspoken veil that was beginning to separate us. Neither one of us wanted to admit that events were beginning to limit us. I could somehow see it in his eyes, and I am sure he saw it in mine.

There is a point in a patient-doctor relationship when both need neutral help to talk about the risks of failure. I could express my feelings to my colleagues—physicians and nurses who knew both of us well. Many of them had worked with me for years and could openly discuss the gigantic problems that faced us. To give Dayem every opportunity to voice his deep concerns, we asked one of our best psychologists to become his confidante. We were worried that Dayem's eagerness to maintain his close relationship to us would leave him no opportunity to express his own anxiety. The veil could become a mutually acceptable barrier of silence that would relieve both of us of the daily discomfort of facing defeat, while permitting a chasm of panic to widen under Dayem's feet.

Physicians are, after all, human. They try consciously or unconsciously to avoid anxiety, and the most anxiety-provoking circumstance for a physician is a growing sense of impotence in the face of an inexorable disease. Patients with chronic disorders like cancer, cystic fibrosis, or thalassemia form a bond with their physicians that is mutually supportive, but it is based on a shared hope for success. When both begin to see that the hope for success is fading, anxiety begins to erode support. Both may seek to avoid anxiety by avoiding the topic. That avoidance creates the veil that descends between them.

One can observe the syndrome of anxiety avoidance most clearly on morning rounds in a hospital. The interns, led by their senior residents, walk around the floor from room to room, examining each patient. Some of the rooms contain patients who will either die on this admission or for whom no known treatment can be effective. Unconsciously, this relatively inexperienced group moves a little faster at such rooms. They hurry their examination and their exchange with the patients as if to rid themselves of the burden; forget about it until tomorrow. Long-term patients who have had many admissions know when that is happening. It is a not-so-subtle message to them that their time is about up. Understandably, they begin to wonder whether the doctor will be there for them when the moment comes.

Much of the training of interns, residents, and nurses needs to be devoted to understanding this dynamic. They are usually young, and the anxiety surrounding impending death is terrible for them. It has a psychological stench that can overwhelm them if they are not supported. Nurses are particularly afflicted. They, after all, spend hour after hour with hospitalized patients, while physicians have brief encounters. Much of the burden of psychologically supporting patients who are facing their mortality falls on nurses, and the burnout frequently seen in young nurses is directly ascribable to the exhaustion that can overcome them from trying to keep their patients' morale, and their own, afloat.

We are fortunate at Children's Hospital. Our nurses seem to find a way to provide remarkable support for patients no matter how much anxiety they feel themselves. It was not at all surprising to me that the nurses flocked to Dayem during this particularly difficult admission. They knew how intelligent he was, how well he must have understood the problems that were facing him, and therefore how frightened he must be. They and the excellent psychologist and some of the young interns and residents did their thing.

I did my best, too, to speak frankly and firmly to him. Together we ripped away the veil. We talked about our concerns and what we were going to do to deal with his problem of access to the circulation. As Dayem had put it, "We would have to try something else."

Soon Dayem went to the operating room for a long operation. The shunt was taken down and replaced with a plastic tubing that ran between the vessels. The tubing could be divided and easily flushed with anticoagulants. We hoped that the flow through the tubing that connected the two vessels would be fast enough to prevent clotting.

With the plastic shunt now in place, we could continue his special transfusions, and using what peripheral veins we could find, we began a two-month constant infusion of Desferal in an attempt to treat his heart failure. Amazingly, Dayem settled his mind to the terribly long hospital stay. Once again, the portable phone was pulled out, and his nimble fingers began punching out telephone numbers that connected him to business opportunities all over the world. He was in constant communication with enterprises, attempting to develop deals while he struggled for the financial and social independence that he so desperately needed. During this admission, the tubing repeatedly clotted, but the clots could be removed, and we had the satisfaction of seeing gram after gram of iron removed by the Desferal.

Finally, just before Christmas of 1983, the moment came for discharge. It had been two admissions and four long months, but Dayem marched out of the hospital free of heart failure, trained to manage his Desferal infusions through the plastic tubing, and full

of promises to take all of his medications, including Desferal, on
schedule, and without failure.

A WEEK AFTER the new year had begun, Dayem was back. The
tubing had clotted again. The clot appeared to extend into the
vein, with obstruction to blood flow in his left leg; his thigh had
begun to swell and had become painful. We opened the plastic tube
and constantly infused the arterial and the venous side with an
anticoagulant for a week until we had achieved excellent flow.
Once again, we sent him back to Washington with our instructions
ringing in his ears.

Whether Dayem was trying to cooperate or not, 1984 was a
ghastly year for him and for all of us, particularly his family, who
were trying to support him. He had no less than ten more hospital
admissions for management of the plastic shunt. No matter what
oral anticoagulants we used, the damnable tubing would clot, neces-
sitating short admissions to clean it out and infuse anticoagulants
directly into the device. Occasionally, the episodes of clotting would
coincide with a scheduled trip to Boston to receive transfusions, but
usually the admissions were unexpected and highly disruptive. It
was impossible for Dayem to lead a normal life; and without some
regularity of schedule and reasonable expectations, it was nearly
impossible for him to develop any confidence in a regular medical
routine, particularly one that involved his own manipulation of the
tubing. Fear of clotting and hospitalization replaced his intense
dislike of the subcutaneous route of administration of Desferal.

The bright spot was Dayem himself. He was clearly beginning
to change his lifestyle. His attention to the details of his medications might have remained irregular, but his interest in his own
future was growing. This was exemplified by his interest in deal-
making and in the growing real estate market in and around Washington. For the first time, he had an office address. It was clear that
Washington-area businessmen were beginning to respect what this
bright and engaging young entrepreneur could do for them. As I
listened to him talk about his ideas, I was tempted to invest in some
of them myself!

The missing piece in Dayem's transformation was his attention to his around-the-clock Desferal schedule. The pump remained a vexing problem. He hated the encumbrance and the inconvenience. He was no longer held back by the adolescent fear of seeming to be different; now it was simply a desire to be free of the trappings of treatment and, above all, to be free of the repeated hospitalizations that were sapping his energy, interrupting progress in his businesses, and disrupting his social life.

I sympathized, but in response to his complaints I kept harping on Dayem to pay strict attention to his treatment and to handle the shunt tubing with exquisite care. In retrospect, I am sure that I was partially blaming him for the episodes of clotting, suggesting that improved compliance would improve the performance of the shunt. "After all," I pointed out, "we put these tubes into many patients, and we just don't have this kind of trouble."

The truth is that Dayem was a uniquely difficult patient for such a treatment. His spleen had been removed, and therefore he had a high platelet count. Platelets are the smallest cells in the blood. They are responsible for the initiation of clotting and are particularly active when they meet a roughened surface. The high platelet count and the roughened surfaces created by the numerous manipulations of the groin vessels certainly contributed to the problem. Dayem *was,* in fact, the cause of the problem, but it wasn't necessarily his personality or his behavior that was responsible. His blood was one important villain. We had to hope that his vessels and the tubing would develop such a smooth surface that the high number of platelets in his blood would eventually glide through the shunt without sticking to it.

Despite our hopes, 1985 was just as bad as the previous year. He had seven more admissions for management of the shunt in addition to his monthly visits for a neocyte-gerocyte exchange. During one of those admissions, we had a long talk about his future in which I began by summarizing all the problems we had to deal with. When I got through with what had to be a rather gloomy inventory, Dayem looked up. "You know, Doc, things could be worse. I have been around this hospital for a long time. I have seen kids in much worse shape than me."

I nodded with admiration.

"I've got a great family. I'm starting to see how I can make some money and be on my own, and you guys have stuck by me. I've got a lot to be grateful for. So cheer up, Doc. You've always said we'll get there; we will."

It was amazing. Here was this young man, confronted by constant transfusions, a devilish plastic contraption in his groin, the threat of heart failure hanging over his head, and *he* was supporting *me!*

"Dayem—you're great—thanks," was all I could say.

"But doc, there is one favor I need you to do for me."

Sensing trouble, I grew wary. "What is it?" I asked.

"Doc, I don't think I really look like a man. Can't you give me some shots?"

Here we go, I thought. He wants testosterone, as if he isn't sexually active enough. Then it hit me in a flash. He'd recently been on a vacation with his family in Monaco. Obviously he had been making invidious comparisons between his short stature and boyish face and the bronzed French playboys ogling the topless girls.

"Dayem," I moaned, "you need testosterone like a cow needs a tuxedo. What are you talking about? Furthermore, testosterone will make you hold on to salt and water, and you're not much better at taking your heart medicine than you are at taking Desferal. If you get testosterone and you don't take heart medicine, you could go into heart failure again."

He looked at me pleadingly.

"Doc, if I can't grow up, I might as well have heart failure."

I stopped arguing and decided to settle the issue by measuring his blood testosterone level. I got him to agree that if the level was normal we would forget about it. Naturally, the level was borderline. Actually, I thought that might be the case. Patients with thalassemia who require regular transfusions often have low or borderline sex hormone levels and remain somewhat sexually underdeveloped even if they live into their twenties. To Dayem's delight, we decided to try a course of hormone replacement. He was pleased to watch his muscles, penis, and body hair grow, but that didn't change his habitual disregard of his other medications.

By the end of 1985, all of us, including Dayem, recognized that the shunt was a failure. There had been too much clotting and infection around the site, surely due to the many maneuvers that had been initiated just to keep it open. We decided on a different approach. First, we took down the shunt in his groin. Then we tunneled a long piece of much smaller plastic tubing under his skin, beginning above his left nipple, and placed the tip of the tubing into a large vessel in his neck. The tubing was then advanced through that neck vein into the largest vein in his chest. There the fast flow should prevent clotting. Through it he could self-infuse Desferal around the clock if he would only do it and if the line did not clot. To our intense frustration, Dayem used the line only intermittently, and there was so such clotting that we were forced to remove it. We had to go back to subcutaneous Desferal if we were to prevent another episode of heart failure.

He returned to Washington full of the usual promises. A few months later, he celebrated his twenty-fourth birthday and kept telling all of us how well he was obeying the rules. But during the summer, it became obvious to us that he was scarcely following any of our instructions.

In the early fall, the roof fell in. Following a particularly hectic week of business and parties, Dayem developed abdominal distension and pain and tenderness in the upper right part of his abdomen. Then he became very short of breath. He again reported to the emergency room at Georgetown Hospital, where he was immediately treated for florid heart failure and sent to us. An extensive cardiac examination confirmed that he had severe iron-related heart muscle damage—so extensive, in fact, that we seriously considered whether this might be his final admission.

I immediately placed a call to his mother, who was then in Paris, to tell her that we had a very serious problem on our hands. It seemed terribly cruel to pile another huge burden onto the many worries about him carried by his mother and his family. But I had no choice—I had to give her the bad news about his heart failure directly and without being able to see her face and watch her response. During that call, I brought her up to date on his treatment; I told her that we had been forced to remove the central line and were again dependent upon subcutaneous Desferal, which Dayem had refused to take, and that he now had another episode of profound heart failure.

Her attitude was very much like her son's.

"We'll have to deal with this too," was her first response. I could almost see her pulling her emotional wagons into a wide circle around her son. She wasn't going to collapse on him and leave him with the task of supporting her as well as himself.

I explained as many of the details to her as I could; Dayem listened to me but could not hear her side of the conversation. Then she asked to speak to him. I gave him the phone and left the room for a while to give them some privacy.

I really don't know exactly what they said to each other. But nearly twenty-five years of trust and support had produced so much faith and determination in both of them that they could emerge from a blow like this without apparent harm. They had a magic touch with each other that pulled away the barbs of sadness and smoothed the painful lacerations they both had to bear. I have seen many children who badly need parental support and who get it with full commitment. But I have never before or since observed as powerful a chemistry as I always see when these two communicate. The bond is so strong that they are almost like the Corsican brothers, one of whom would feel pain when the other was injured. On several occasions I would receive a call from Mrs. Saif at a particularly difficult time when the shunt or the long central line was clogging. From thousands of miles away, she had sensed trouble and was calling to check on the circumstance.

This time she simply threw herself into the emotional breach, and by letting Dayem know that she would always be there for him, she gave him the confidence to move ahead.

When I returned to see him, he displayed his optimistic view. "There is no point looking back, doc. I've been like this before. You'll get me out of it."

"Maybe," I muttered to myself grimly. We had been able to rescue quite a few patients like this with careful cardiac management and weeks of intravenous Desferal, but we had never done it twice in one patient, and this was Dayem's second episode of major cardiac failure. Would this immortal sword make it through another disaster?

Two months later the answer was positive. We had hooked him up to continuous intravenous Desferal, carefully titrated his cardiac drugs, and inserted another long central line for home therapy. He would triumphantly march back to Washington again—to his deals, his real estate business, and his endless parties—full of promises and praise for us. "Doc, you guys did a good job," he began.

"Dayem, never mind the good job stuff. Stop buttering me up—are you going to stay out of here or are you going to ignore the program and wind up moving in here for the rest of your life?"

"Doc, I understand. Take it easy. It will all work out."

With that, he was back in the fast lane.

THOUGH I FULLY expected him to return promptly with another episode of heart failure, I was surprised. On his next check-up all of our tests showed that he must have had enough of a scare to cooperate. His iron levels were quite decent, and the levels of cardiac drugs were reasonable as well. We praised him and sent him on his way.

He was out on his own for six entire months, until just before his twenty-fifth birthday. Then the central line clotted and could not be reopened. We tried everything, including an attempt to pass a wire through the tubing. I don't like that procedure because of the risk that the wire may break through the tubing and puncture a large vessel, but we tried it because we did not want to be forced to put him through another central line replacement.

After a few hours of struggle, we gave up and replaced the line for the third time. He bounced out of the hospital in four days and returned briefly only twice—two months and then seven months later—for treatment of infections around the central line site. Naturally, we were convinced that he had not managed the central line with enough care and insisted that he follow through on every detail of the procedure. He would look at us with the practiced eye of a man who had listened to these bores for a few too many years.

Our constant hectoring must have had some effect, however, because Dayem remained out of the hospital for nearly a year. He did not return to visit in our beds until three months after his twenty-sixth birthday, when the central line failed again. In fact, it had broken in the tunnel under the skin. We replaced it for the fourth time and took advantage of the admission to perform some sophisticated heart studies. To our amazement and his delight, his exercise tolerance was quite normal, and his heart rate, rhythm, and blood pressure responses to exercise were excellent. Dayem looked particularly mischievous after those tests.

"You see, doc, I told you not to worry. I'll be fine. Just let me do things my own way."

"Dayem, if I let you do things your way, you and your buddies would get us all arrested by the vice squad."

He roared with laughter. "Oh doc, we've had quite a time together, but give me some credit. I really did pay attention, and look at the result. The figures don't lie, and I don't lie either."

"You did much better, Dayem, but for God's sake, keep it up. We just can't go through this again. The next heart failure could be your last. You can see what the Desferal can do for you if you only take it."

Whether it was some as yet undetermined change in the tendency of his blood to coagulate, better technique on his part, the will of God, or a combination of all three, Dayem turned a remarkable corner in 1988 and 1989.

He was admitted only three times in 1989. The first admission occurred two months after his twenty-seventh birthday because a special study showed some deterioration in the strength of the beat of his heart. This, we were convinced, was due to his carelessness about his Desferal dose and his heart medications. We tuned him up for a few days in July and discharged him with our usual warnings. He returned for a check-up with a sunny smile and beguiling promises. He even wore a T-shirt bearing the inscription *Moderation*. He bought it, he said, in preference to one marked *Abstinence*.

That fall, he had another episode of infection at the site of entry of the central line into his skin. The infection was easily managed with antibiotics.

His third admission was just before Christmas of 1989 for the same problem, and he required a week of intensive antibiotic therapy to resolve it. Except for a tunnel infection in 1995, Dayem Saif has not darkened our inpatient doors since January 1990. We see him regularly, of course, for his neocyte-gerocyte exchanges. But incredibly, he has stayed away from the beds, turning his full attention to his business and social life.

He is remarkably adept in business. He had begun his career at the age of seventeen with his bullet-proof limousine sales to wealthy Near East potentates. He earned $80,000 in that business, before his father made him discontinue the trade because he considered it dishonorable. Dayem asked him what was dishonorable about $80,000, but he dutifully abandoned the business and entered hospital equipment sales. That turned out to be less than rewarding, and so he began selling construction material all over the world, borrowing money from banks to buy the materials and selling them abroad. His company became very successful, and at the age of twenty-four he established a biotechnology company that developed and sold cancer diagnostics and special blood tubes for transporting body fluids for analysis. That too became profitable. At age twenty-nine he established an Italian restaurant in the Washington suburbs. Here again he was quickly successful. He has an uncanny eye for what will work and a smart head for calculating a profit margin. He also has intense family loyalty. His brothers joined his businesses, and they work together with complete compatibility.

"We've got no secrets, Doc, in our family. We stick together, and we're loyal to each other. That really works in business."

Shortly before Dayem's twenty-eighth birthday, his younger brother was married in a big wedding held in Paris. It was a tremendous party, and Dayem was there in full cry for a good time. I imagined how his family must have felt. Twenty-two years before, he had left Europe on *The France*, a sickly, pale, tiny boy who had broken nearly every bone in his body. Now he returned as a successful young businessman and *bon vivant*. True, he had plenty of problems, some of them extraordinarily serious; but he had mastered them in his mind, and he danced the night away to celebrate his brother's new-found happiness.

He wrote a brief note to me from France.

Dear Doc, Don't worry so much about me. I am a survivor, but
thank you for worrying anyway.
  Love always, Dayem

The note was written with a strong hand. It was Dayem to a T, but his intermittent noncompliance continued. On a winter vacation in southern France, he *forgot* his heart medication for a week and returned having gained five pounds of fluid. We were all furious and fought with him. He apologized and agreed with us. It was the same old performance. As soon as he resumed his medication schedule, he greatly improved. A month later the line clogged, and we removed a solid deposit of Desferal from it. Obviously, he had failed to flush the line carefully, as his instructions demanded. Again, I flew into a rage. Again, he promised to be faithful to the program. Again, we shook hands, and again, he disappeared into his very enjoyable and now lucrative life.

On his twenty-ninth birthday, little had changed. He was more active than ever in business, and enjoying himself no end.

"Doc, one day I'll be rich, and I'll give this hospital a million dollars. Just wait and see," he said.

"Dayem, I'd practically pay *you* a million dollars if you'd just find the time to take care of yourself."

"Doc, you take things too seriously. Just relax. Things will be fine. Wait and see." Later that day, he confessed that he didn't take any medication very regularly. "Doc, it's hard to remember to take pills. I'm busy, you know."

So much for an oral iron chelator that has to be taken with high frequency. If he couldn't remember digitalis, how could he remember any drug that would have to be taken at least every four hours? I often caution my colleagues that we won't necessarily improve compliance in many adolescents even if we find an orally active iron remover unless the drug can be designed so that it needs to be taken only once or at most twice a day. Even then, I wonder if most adolescents will really take it faithfully.

By Christmas of 1991 we were becoming very concerned again. His iron levels were up, and his cardiac function was down. Again,

Desferal compliance was the critical issue. So immediately after the new year, we had a high-level conference. The three physicians and the nurse responsible for his care crammed into a little office in the transfusion service with him, and I began the litany. "Dayem, here we go again. You know what this is all about." He was dressed in blue jeans and a fashionable leather jacket, and I had to admit that he looked wonderful.

"Doc, you know I really do hear you. I know what all of you think. You look at my heart and my blood and my iron and my pills, and you see *those things*. I see my business and my friends and my family. Doc, you know, I never thought I'd even have a business and friends and a girlfriend. And here I am. I don't want to think about the other stuff too much. I just want to get on with my life. I can't stop to worry about lines and pills and Desferal."

I opened my mouth to speak, but he raised his hand.

"Doc, I know what you're going to say. I have been listening for almost twenty-five years. I know you love me, and I know you want the best for me. And before you say anything, I am really going to promise you that I'll get in great shape for you."

"Not for me, Dayem. For you."

"Doc, whichever way you want it, I'll get in shape for both of us. How's that? Then we'll have a party. OK?"

Incredibly, we were rapidly approaching his thirtieth birthday. If he would only take his medications regularly, we could make that celebration and have more years to spare.

Who, I wondered, would have believed that he would actually reach the age of thirty? I could still see him in our clinic on his first visit—frail, anemic, and close to heart failure. Yet, here he was—successful and very much alive, if miserably frustrating. What a celebration that thirtieth birthday would be!

Celebration
and Reflection

THE NOTION that we might organize a surprise thirtieth birthday party for Dayem occurred to me as I was talking to him
that day in the transfusion service. I became convinced that we *had*
to celebrate his day. Together we had accomplished the impossible,
and we deserved a party—everyone who had helped our Immortal
Sword to survive: doctors, nurses, blood bank technicians, and,
above all, his family. The task was to plan it successfully and keep
the secret from him. Fortunately, my birthday falls on the same day
as his. I casually invited him to come to my house after his next
transfusion to celebrate my birthday, and he accepted. "Don't be
late," I cautioned. "Be there exactly at 6:00 p.m. Jean is very
punctual, you know." He promised faithfully (as he always does)
that he would be there and precisely on time.

The door bell rang promptly at five. I was still trying to get my
necktie in place and stabbed at it hopelessly. The thin end came out
much longer than the wide one and I gave up in disgust. The door
bell rang again insistently.

"It must be the nurses," I called to Jean as she pulled a brush
through her hair, "they're always on time."

"Well, answer the door; we can't leave them out there just
ringing the bell."

With the thin end of my tie dangling foolishly and feeling
incompletely prepared, I hurried downstairs, answered the door,
and confirmed my prediction. The nurses had arrived all together

and absolutely on time. I greeted them affectionately as the good friends they are, but I had to ask them how they do it.

"You folks are never late. Every time we plan a conference or even a party, you're always ready at the appointed hour. Doctors are never on time. Is it biological or environmental? It's not gender because female doctors are never on time either."

They looked a bit uncomfortable, noticed my tie, and apologized for being prompt.

"You see, WE have things to do on a schedule. You'll never really understand." We looked at one another and burst out laughing. We had worked together for so long that we knew and rather liked our various foibles, and this was a moment we had eagerly awaited for months. We had planned the surprise party for Dayem together, and in the process we had assigned duties quite carefully. A surprise party can only work if all the guests arrive before the surprised one, if the guest of honor actually arrives at all, if the entire company of partygoers has a lot in common, and if the food is good. We had it all worked out, but I had some concerns.

I adjusted my tie, this time under the watchful view of Dorothy Patton, the nurse manager. Of course the tie came out perfectly just as the door bell rang again. Incredibly, all of the physicians entered together; the chief of immunology, the Blood Bank staff, and a young hematologist now responsible for direct supervision of Dayem's treatment. With them were my children and their spouses. The bell rang for the third time. Dayem's family had made it from all parts of the world—all of them together! It was incredible. I muttered a thankful Ins'Allah (God willing). We had everyone! Then I thanked the nurses and Cathy Lantigua, my indomitable assistant who had made it all happen. The party began while we waited for Dayem and gaily renewed old friendships.

I kept looking at my watch nervously. Where was Dayem? Suddenly, through the window, I spied a car in the driveway. Dayem and his girlfriend climbed out dressed in their finest. He smiled warmly as I opened the door. "Hi Doc," was his standard greeting.

"Doc, I almost forgot, Happy Birthday to you."

"But Dayem, this is your birthday too—and a big one—your thirtieth. We should be celebrating your birthday more than mine."

He smiled his huge smile and looked at me affectionately. "So we'll celebrate together, you and I."

He looked marvelous. He had none of the pasty brown color of previous years. Though a bit shorter than an average American and slight of build, he appeared almost debonair in his English-cut blue suit, white shirt, and Italian tie.

"Come on into the living room, Dayem, we'll wait for Jean in there."

As we crossed the front hall into the living room, Dayem's mouth fell open in amazement. Arrayed before him were his mother, his two brothers, one with his new bride and the other with a girlfriend, my wife and children, my administrative assistant, the physicians who had cared for him, and the nurses in the Blood Bank and in the Clinical Research Center who had seen him through the past twenty-five years. With a single deafening chorus they all cried out "HAPPY BIRTHDAY, DAYEM!"

He was stunned, totally surprised, and terribly happy and proud. He grasped and hugged everyone one at a time, looked at them with such sincere fondness that tears came to my eyes. Then he walked over to me, put his arms around me, and said, "Thank you, Doc." When I hugged him, I felt the pump in its holster under his right arm.

"And Dayem, you're wearing the damned pump! You're actually still doing what you're supposed to do!"

"Doc, would I let you down on your birthday?"

A FEW HOURS later when everyone had departed, Dayem and I sat down to talk. I could see that there were many issues on his mind, and I asked his permission to tape-record our conversation so that I could recall the details. He agreed, and the following is nearly a verbatim transcript of what he had to say.

"Happy Birthday, Doc. It was a wonderful party—thank you. You know there are some things I've never told you. First of all, you've often wondered what I remember about myself. Well, two distinctive things happened. I had two unique dreams; one when I was five and one when I was six. When I was five, I guess as a way to explain to myself everything that was going on, I had this incredible dream where I was seeing myself almost as though I was a wide-angle lens. I was in a nursery with all these other babies. I had just been born, and I was with all these other babies, and I was one of them. And I was picked by God to die—to be with him out of all these babies, and it was an honor. And at the last minute, it was decided that I wasn't going to die, and I was put back. That was the first dream, and that was when I was five years old.

"Then when I was six, I had this dream where there was an old man with a white beard sitting on a throne; you know, a child's image of God, and he said, 'Dayem, don't be scared. I am God, and from now on, everything's going to be all right.' From then on, everything *has* been all right; that's really what's happened to me, and that dream when I was six is what's made me survive everything that I have survived with this almost arrogant air that everything is going to be all right. When I was a child I was being truly picked upon because kids can be very, very vicious, about my looks, about the way that I was, about the fact that they were told by the teacher that they couldn't play with me because they would hurt me. It wasn't all their fault, but I was picked upon continuously at school. You know; I was called Bugs Bunny and I was called this and that, and I remember kids used to tell me, 'Why do you look this way? Why are you this way?' and I said, 'Because God made me that way, and if you don't like it, tough.' I mean these dreams made me think I was a saint and that's what gave me this inner strength that made me tolerate everything and basically made me continue and not give up and not hide my head in the sand, which is what a lot of people would have done in the same circumstances.

"Years later I had forgotten all about these dreams. I was sitting down in a restaurant with my mother, and she said, 'Do you remember those two dreams?' Then it hit me. The dreams were true. If you recall, I was six when I came to see you, and that's exactly when everything started being all right, when I started getting better, when the fractures were less, and I began to live. So that has always stayed with me, that basic spirituality, if you will, and that, I think, is the most important thing that I remember.

"It was so difficult for me to make friends at the beginning. I was a six-year-old in Mexico when I went to my first school. I had never made a friend before that. It was an incredible lesson. For example, the first lesson I ever learned was to laugh at myself. I learned that when I did something wrong in first grade. The punishment for somebody that did something wrong in first grade was to go in front of the class of kindergartners, wearing a pacifier. This was supposed to be the punishment. So I went in front of kindergarten, wearing a pacifier, and I started cracking up laughing, and then the whole class started laughing, and so it wasn't really a punishment. I got the best out of the whole situation.

"But, throughout my childhood, I felt odd-looking. Well I *knew* I was odd-looking. I always knew I was odd-looking because I was constantly *told* I was odd-looking. My whole life I was told I was odd-looking, but it was never terrible. It was never something that injured me or hurt me tremendously, my looks, because I made friends, and I was accepted, and it was okay, but I always wanted to look better if I could, and then I wanted to look better because of girls more than anything else. I think that was really why I wanted to look better. After having the operation on my face, I was told by my best friend, 'I couldn't tell you this before, but at some times, I was embarrassed to take you to parties because of the way that you looked even though you were my best friend.'

"And at that time, I never really had any girls. I was every girl's confidante. I was almost every boy's confidante too. That was my forte. People could talk to me about anything, and a lot of times I would solve their problems. I was like the class psychologist. My first love was this girl who was from Mexico City, the daughter of my parents' best friends. They had three daughters, and my parents had three sons. We used to take trips together, and I was in love with the oldest girl. Of course, she was never in love with me and had nothing to do with me, but she was my best friend so she would tell me about all her problems. So that was my first love, but I always knew that there wasn't a relationship there, that she didn't feel the same way about me that I felt about her, and it was puppy love anyway. It was a childish love. I liked girls, but I never really had a girlfriend when I was in high school. I never really did. Instead I had those Desferal shots.

"When I came here, and they gave me the first shot, I don't think you knew what the dosage ought to be, and it was excruciatingly painful. And I remember that I think I was in tears from the shot, and then I was told that I had to have it every day, which made me more upset. But in the end the shots were okay. My mother used to give them to me when we were in Mexico, and then when we went to London, I got this gun, and I did it myself, and I liked the whole idea of giving myself a shot. After a while, I threw away the gun and just did it by hand, and the shot was okay.

"I gave them to myself in my legs and thighs. I used to alternate. You know, one time this leg, one time the other leg. That was okay, and then we started on the pump. I remember it used to be an almost half a kilo pump, and I used to have to put a needle under the skin on my stomach, and it wasn't comfortable, but I remember I wore it every day twenty-four hours a day. I used to wear it in class and you know people used to push the red button. There used to be a red button that gives you a flush. You know, it was like a cool thing. I turned it into something exciting, and then what happened was I got an infection with 15 milliliters of pus, and I think that really turned me off the pump totally. Of course it was always bothering me and irritating my skin, and produced bumps on my skin, but on top of that I had an infection, and it was awful.

"Afterwards, it really was cramping my style. Afterwards, it was taking away from that little bit of freedom that I had. I couldn't swim when others wanted to swim, I couldn't do this when the other ones wanted to do that. It was cumbersome. It was annoying. It was painful. It itched. It was no fun. It really wasn't any fun whatsoever. And it wasn't anything that I was making up because I didn't want to wear it, it just wasn't comfortable. If it was more comfortable, I think it might have been different. I would have found a way to make it okay, but it really wasn't.

"So by the time I got to Washington, I was really not about to use that pump. That's why I had so many discussions about it with you, Doc. I was using it some. I just wasn't using it the way that I was supposed to be using it. To be honest, I wasn't using it at all.

In a way, it was unfortunate that I was smart enough to know what the numbers meant—to know the liver and the heart numbers and to know what they meant. I knew that I wasn't really in immediate danger, and so I thought whether I skipped a year or two wasn't going to make much difference in the long run.

"So I told myself that everything was fine. Two years was not going to make a difference, and on top of all that, I was being told that I might die anyway, and that the Desferal was not necessarily something that was going to get me out of trouble. So that's why in a way that I thought that it would be all right if I skipped it. And remember, I never let myself get beyond a certain point. In other words, whenever I realized that I was sick, I came back. I stayed in the hospital for two months at a time. I got a shunt. I got a central line. I got this; I got that. So I think that at one point even though you thought that I had suicidal tendencies, and you even wanted me to see a psychologist, and I saw him a few times, I stopped seeing him because I basically told him whatever I wanted to tell him and whatever I thought he wanted to hear, and because he wasn't doing anything for me, himself, or for anybody, though he was a very nice man.

"You know, I always knew one thing. My big point was *not* to die. My point was to live my life the fullest that I could live it within the margins that I gave myself that I thought were permissible. You know when I thought I crossed that line, then right away I got back on the program, and whatever I had to do, whether it was sacrificing two months of my life in the hospital or something else, I did it because I knew that was the only way, and I didn't want to die. You know I still don't want to die. I have no intention of doing so.

"The other belief that has helped me through is the certainty I feel that there is a plan for me. Whose plan is it? Well, I'm the first to admit that it's not just a divine plan. It's certainly not just my plan. And it's not just your plan either. It's a bit of everything. When you would scare me to death, that had something to do with it. That made me do certain things. When my mother would tell me, 'Well, we trust you, and we're behind you and whatever you want, we'll do,' well, that had something to do with it. So it was nobody's specific plan. It was the work of everybody, synergy, something put together by everybody that has really carried me this far.

"Doc, do you remember when I had encephalitis or meningitis? I was in my room upstairs on the third floor, vomiting automatically, half-conscious, half not-conscious, my eyes totally paralyzed so I couldn't look to the right or the left, I could only see in front of me; my neck was killing me because of the swelling of the brain. I remember my father carrying me down the stairs with my mother behind. It was terribly painful, and I was put in the back of the limousine, and they were sitting in the bucket seats of the limousine, and the driver was driving. I could only see the roof of the car, obviously, I couldn't see anything else, and I remember the driver went to the wrong entrance of NIH from where he was supposed to go, and then all of a sudden, he tells my parents, 'It's closed. This is not the right place. What do we do?' So I said, 'Go backwards, turn left, turn right, go this way, go that way,' and I directed him, half-consciously, to the door of the NIH where we were supposed to go and where there were people waiting for us to arrive. Somehow I could do all that even though I was only half-conscious.

"I remember that the next day, all my friends came, and my parents were there, and I had this feeling that I wasn't going to die. I just knew it. I knew it within me that I wasn't going to die. I remember I cried. I cried for an hour or so with my mother, and it was the most incredible thing. I remember crying with her, 'Oh my God, I'm not going to die, but I'm going to be paralyzed. Where are the cyanide pills? What are we going to do? I am not going to die, but I'm going to be paralyzed.' And, of course, a month later, I was water skiing and I was totally recovered—an incredible recovery. And nobody really knew why it came or why it didn't come and what it really was, but that changed my life. That incident changed my life. It changed my way of thinking about things. Just before that incident I was very destructive, very crazy, doing a lot of stupidities, and I think that in a way the illness made me mature just a little bit. It made me start changing my way of life for a way that was healthier and better.

"And now I feel so normal that, apart from coming here every three weeks and getting some blood, my life is not that affected. I have a steady girlfriend so I am not worried about having a central line on my chest. You know you can play tic-tac-toe on my chest with all the scars that I have. So it's not a problem of vanity anymore. I am just not that affected by my disease. It's not a problem, and it never was because I never hid it. I never hid it from anybody. I never tried to hide the fact that I was sick. I never tried to hide the fact that I had thalassemia. I never tried to deny it. In fact, it was something that I used to my benefit. When I was a little kid, I used to use the pump to get into movies where only kids who were eighteen or older were allowed. I was sixteen but I looked like twelve, and I would get into a movie where I wasn't supposed to get in because I said, 'I am sick, and that's why I look younger than what I really am, and here's the pump.' Or if there was a restaurant with a two-hour waiting line, I would go to the person there and say, 'Listen, I am out of the hospital, I only have two hours to eat, and could you get us a table?' 'Oh sure, no problem.' We'd have a party of six with all my friends, and we'd be seated. So, on the contrary, I always used it to my benefit. So, it's never really been that much of a problem.

"One of my biggest problems was the time when I was reaching puberty around sixteen. Everybody was so happy that I reached puberty because they felt that I might not. But what happened was that I reached puberty, and then it stopped. And that created a lot of problems in me because my testosterone was not at the normal level. Mentally, I liked girls because I had always liked girls, but physically I didn't have the libido if you will, and I wasn't as interested as other kids, and I truly started worrying that maybe I was a homosexual, and also because people used to make fun of me—you know the way I walked was slightly effeminate, the way I appeared was odd, and I really, really truly worried because I knew that I wasn't a homosexual, yet I wasn't sure, and this was a big problem for me and caused me a lot of anguish—the not knowing, the bizarreness, the thoughts that would go across my head. And then when I realized that I had a low testosterone level, then it was all explained to me.

"You see, I made certain about sex. When I was young, I told myself that I would do certain things by a certain age. I set goals for myself. So by the age of sixteen, I was going to make love to a woman no matter who it was, and I was going to have a girlfriend. I was going to have all the things that I didn't have that other kids had, and I reached all my goals. Well, the first time I had sex was with a prostitute, but then, when I lived in Washington, I was seventeen and a half, and there was this girl, and she became my girlfriend, and she fell madly in love with me, and we went out for four years and had sex all the time, and everything was fine because of the goal. But even with that relationship, I had in the back of my mind the thought that things were not exactly right within me physically, and I didn't know what it was. It disturbed me a lot, and I really never talked to anybody about it. I kept it mostly to myself, and it was very hard. And then when I started with the hormone treatments, that changed. All of that changed, and it helped me a lot. So I don't know if it's because of the severe iron overload that I wasn't producing enough testosterone or what the real reason was for it, or if it was just because of the thalassemia, but I had a great complex, you know, a penis complex. I always thought my penis was too small. So I was very complex sexually, but I was complex in every other way, too, and yet I surpassed almost everything. But the sexual issue was a great struggle within me. It was a great frustration within me. It caused me to feel a lot of shame.

"Doc, you've often asked me how I deal with everything now in my life and why I've improved so much in the past three years. I'm convinced that the change is due to meditation and metaphysics. It's a philosophy that's been around for thousands of years, and it's one that says that you create your own reality. It means that everything that happens in your life happens because you allow it to happen or you want it to happen. Let me give you an example. Until three years ago my business was terrible. I couldn't close a deal to save my life. I formed a company. We had a contract, a million dollar contract, to supply building materials for a project, and we were one of three bidders. We won the bid, we had everything done, we had a nice margin of profit, we went to the Gulf, we signed the contract, and the guy goes bankrupt. So the deal falls through. I convinced my uncle to invest for himself with a guy that I was involved with in real estate, and the guy never returned the money. I mean just one problem after another, just one disaster after another.

"And then I realized by meditation that I was getting into these lousy deals because I actually wanted to feel the shame that I had never let myself feel. It was the shame that came from childhood, that came from when I was abandoned in a subtle way by my father because in his eyes, because of his religion, because of his way of looking at life, he deals with tragedy by saying it is done, it is written. Deep in him, he believed that it was written by God that I would die, and he dealt with it by accepting it. In a way, I was written off. I wasn't loved any less. He loves me very much. It was just his way of dealing with it. But that, nonetheless, was a form of abandonment, and that abandonment instilled shame in me, and shame is not a matter of the difference between wrong or right. Shame is being a mistake itself. It's being a wrong person, not just committing a wrong act. That sense of shame continued in my childhood when I was being told that I looked funny, when I was being told that I was different, when I was being told that I was weak.

"On top of the shame of being insulted, there was the shame that my own body in a way betrayed me because it was not working. It was not doing what it was supposed to do. It was not growing. It was breaking itself. It was sick, and created more of the shame which I never allowed myself to feel when I was young. If I felt it, I would have been devastated. I rose above the shame, but the force of that shame was still inside of me, and it was still doing something in me, and that's why I created these incidents that might let me feel the shame. Going, for example, to a casino, having no money and losing a crazy amount of money that I didn't have was a way to feel the incredible shame that was within me. But I wouldn't feel it, I would laugh it off. Then an inner voice would say, 'Oh, you don't want to feel it this time, well you have another chance!' Then I would make another and bigger terrible incident and then bigger and bigger and bigger, and you can see it, can't you? When I realized what I was doing, and I could see it, 'My

God, this really is happening.' When I was able to realize through meditation that that's what it was, and I was able to feel the shame in meditation and *really* feel the inner shame and be rid of it, everything changed. My first deal came. I paid all my debts. I didn't owe anybody anything. Business deals are going like they never went before, and now everything goes automatically almost in a magical way.

"I often ask myself, 'Why would God or any force create a life-threatening, inherited blood disease?' There's no real scientific explanation. I mean yes, it's inherited, but there's no real logical way that you could explain it. Actually, it has saved me. If I really knew that by being born of my particular father and mother, from that inheritance, that I would have to live somewhere around the Persian Gulf; that I would have to follow in my father's footsteps; that I would have had to be under that type of social situation, I would have never been able to survive. I have survived this disease much more than I could have survived that life, and this disease has given me the excuse to live the way that I want to live, to do everything that I have wanted to do without anybody being able to have input into me such as, 'Well, why aren't you here?' or 'Why aren't you doing this?' or 'Why isn't he here?' I had the best excuse in the world. So in a way it was a very ingenious way of getting out of my situation.

"Unfortunately, I put myself in a different jail which is this jail of bad health which metaphysically I am trying to get out of, and in the past three years since I have started with this way of thinking, I have been getting out of my health jail. There is no way, for example, to explain why my heart numbers are better now than they were in the past five years. And I am getting older. My numbers are incredible. I'm healthier than I've ever been. I haven't even had a cold in I don't know how long when I used to have one every month.

"Now, doc, I don't want to go *too* far into all this, but a lot of things in metaphysics make a lot of sense and I can tell you that meditation saved me.

"You know, there is a higher being—call it God, call it Jehovah, you know, whatever you want to call it, but there is a God that only wants love, that only *is* love, that only wants us to be happy and to experience joy, and not the God you've been told about; the God who says, 'You have to work hard and you have to suffer and you have to be happy with what you have and so on and so forth,' which doesn't make sense. God is above judging. We judge ourselves. I think we are the hardest judges of all. You want to give somebody a punishment, tell the person to define the punishment. People will give themselves the worst punishment that you could think of for them; I think that that's what happens when we judge ourselves. I don't believe anymore in brutal self-judgment, and I've been learning not to do that—not to live with shame for the past three years. Now I just try to deal with all of my life, not just my health, but everything, and it's helped. I'm convinced that's why I don't have so many clots and infections and why I can take my medicines as I'm supposed to.

"Deep in my heart, I don't think that thalassemia is going to kill me. Whether it does or it doesn't really doesn't matter that much anymore to me. I am satisfied and happy with my life with the way that I am, with the things that I'm doing and with knowing that there's something more. In other words, I feel strong enough, confident enough, that there is more to life than life itself. So if I happen to die, it's okay. I really won't die. It's just my body that will die. I will continue.

"As I said before, I used to use my disease for my benefit, and I have done that my whole life, and now I have to stop doing that because in a way that's why I'm holding on to it—why I won't let go of it. Let's assume for a second that I could even let go of the disease. It's part of my personality right now so even if I could, it's not an easy thing to do because it's part of me, and it's been part of me for so long; it's part of my story. It's part of what makes me interesting. It's like, 'Hi, I'm Dayem. This disease is me.' If I got rid of all this, well, who would I really be? So it's quite strange, but I am trying to let go of that part as much as I can. And the way that I'm trying to let go of it the most that I can is by not martyring myself, for example, by not taking my medicines, by things of that sort. So it all goes around in a circle. Even though I should be able to just will it away, I can't just say, 'Well, I am going to will it away and not do anything for it.' And I have to continue doing everything for it that I'm supposed to do. But that's how I deal with it basically.

"I've learned something else, too, Doc. I've learned how to relate to you and the hospital. You know the hospital is an integral part of me. I mean I have a totally different outlook about doctors and hospitals than anybody in the world has. I can walk into a hospital anywhere and know where everything is. I know exactly who to go to. I walk in like I'm a doctor myself, which is very strange for other people. You know, when most people go to a hospital themselves, it's a frightening thing. For me, it's second nature. It's like being at home. But the relationship with the doctors—I've gone through a lot of relationships, and they've all been very nice. They have all been very touching. They've all been very close. There have been mutual feelings between me and all the doctors and nurses who I've had experience with, and they all have a genuine care, which is nice. I mean it's a genuine care, it's not just, you know, smiles and, 'Oh God, he's here again.' It's genuine, and you can see it, and you can feel it, and it's nice.

"I know I was very sick when you first saw me. I have no idea of what your thoughts must have been. For me it would be totally different because I have gone through it. I don't know how someone who hasn't gone through what I have gone through would think about a kid who looked like me when I was six. I mean I guess it must have been a feeling of, 'Let's see what we can do, and let's do the best we can.' I don't know how much more you could feel right away before you have a real bond. I mean what can a doctor feel at the beginning? You've told me that you had never seen anybody walk into a clinic that sick—that it was an extraordinary event. You wondered whether you were going to get me upstairs before I died right there in the clinic. That's incredible from two points of view. For me, it's incredible that being that sick, I was still walking, and I was still laughing, and I was still talking. For you, it's more like, 'My God, he's going to die any moment. What are we going to do?' And I think that that's the difference between the doctor and the patient. All I had to make sure of was that I was walking and doing whatever I could to be alive!

"It's great for me to realize now that I had the strength to make it—that you've never before seen somebody walking in with the hemoglobin level that I had. I mean it almost makes me proud. It makes me believe that there is a higher power watching over me. It makes me feel good to think that, and I think there is a higher power. I am sure there is. After all, there's a lot we cannot explain. I certainly can't explain why the last three years have gone so well. You've told me that there is no clear scientific basis for that. Nothing has changed. The last piece of tubing we put in was no better than the first. The last three years have been so successful that I truly believe that future years will get better and better. I'm going to make it, Doc. We'll celebrate our birthdays together from now on."

WHEN Dayem ceased talking, we sat there together silently for a while. For the first time I was beginning to understand what had occurred during the past three years. His improvement with respect to clotting and infection around the central line had been, up to this time, inexplicable. Now I had a glimmer of insight. The coagulation mechanism is highly responsive to emotional control. This is an important survival mechanism. Wounded and frightened animals have very high levels of platelets and certain plasma clotting factors. These responses help the animals to staunch the flow of blood. Several experiments, conducted in normal, healthy volunteers, have demonstrated the stimulatory effect of anxiety on human clotting function.

In the absence of a better explanation, I have to conclude that Dayem's adoption of meditation reduced his level of anxiety, and this in turn may have induced his clotting factors to fall to a level that permitted him to co-exist with the central line. Freedom from anxiety also permitted him to accept the daily duties involved in compliance with his medication schedule. As he had come to know himself and gain self-respect, he had pushed aside a huge load of doubt, shame, and anxiety and had instead found a way to live with his disease without permitting it to dominate him.

Families, Patients, and Doctors

T HE DAY AFTER THE PARTY, and that long soliloquy by Dayem, I decided to visit with Mrs. Saif. What, I wondered, had impressed her most over the course of her son's chronic illness? Had her attitude, her values, her family changed during the past thirty years of almost unremitting stress? Here are some of her thoughts, which I recorded.

"I was only twenty-five when this began and I must admit that I started with great bitterness. Perhaps I never told you that a doctor advised me to accept the fact that I had only one child. I did not accept it. My body did not accept it. My mind and heart did not accept it. I had *two* children at the time. When that doctor told me, 'Consider you only have one child,' it was an insult to my mother-hood, to me as a human being. I took it very personally. It was not because I couldn't believe that Dayem might die, but I wouldn't let anyone condemn him before he was really ready to die. Yes, had he died a day later, *then* I would have considered I had only one child. But at that moment, I was not ready to consider that disaster. I had two children. I kept saying to myself, they are here, they are here, they are here.

"Immediately after I came to this hospital, knowing you and everybody who was committed to Dayem, I grew up quickly. Some-how instead of being a twenty-five-year-old person, I became sixty all of a sudden and in a very nice way. Yes, I became sixty—I understood the world, understood that this is not the end of the world, that there are so many other people who are much worse off. One should not be egocentric and just look at oneself as being the center of the world. There are other people, other things, other problems, and when a problem can be dealt with, it's not a problem anymore; it becomes a search for a solution. That's how I lived through it, I guess.

"Later was the phase of gratitude. I feel so enriched by everything that has happened. I sometimes look at myself, at what I could have become without Dayem's disease. I would be a stupid, good-looking woman who lives in an environment of receptions and dinner parties. My husband's business requires constant entertaining and dealing with people at a level that is totally superficial. I know the women who live that life. I talk to them. They are my friends. They see life in a different way, and they are very happy. That's fine, but I don't want to be them, and I would have most probably become them without Dayem. So that's why I have gratitude to him. He freed me. So to me, the good that has come from this is much, much bigger than the bad.

"Yes, Dayem suffered a lot, but he has also become a different person because of his suffering. He is a sharer and giver—he's a joy. Even when he has to give me bad news on the phone, we manage to laugh our heads off with that bad news, feeling most awful, but still seeing the humor of it. I've learned to look at catastrophe in a different way. I mean it's a bit like Jewish humor. You know, you find the funny thing in despair. You understand the humorous part of a situation. Jews call it the practice of despair, but I would call it even more than that. It's not despair any more when you can see it from another angle that makes it a much smaller thing because you can see it in perspective.

"Furthermore, we've both learned not to peer too far into the future. We are living our lives. He's thirty, and he is living his own life. He is doing his business. He is happy. We don't live together anymore, but we are in very close touch. The love, the caring, the humor is still there, and we can speak on the phone every single day or stay for a month without speaking on the phone. Whenever we speak, the relationship is exactly the same, and he knows that if he wants something, he can find me, and I know if I want something, I can find it with him. We live everyday, we live it today. We live this minute. I don't think anymore of death. Who isn't going to die? Whoever told us that our children would not die? I mean, when someone says, 'Your child is going to die'—the reaction is to say, 'Oh my God!' But, really, that's an obvious statement, after all. One's child might have an accident. Nobody gives us a lease for 450 years. The thing is to live the second, the day, the year, and enjoy it and get it at its best and just try to be yourself. I know I don't have a lease on life—on his life or mine or anybody else's. Every second is a gift, and I cherish that gift. I am grateful. That's how I feel with Dayem. He is a link to the best I can be. And, you know, he plays that role with many different people.

"When all that stress about Dayem's refusal to take his medication was going on, I'm sure my two healthy sons suffered. I'm sure that at one time or another they have had mixed feelings: all children do. I mean they must have thought that number one is taking our mother's time, and her complete attention and focus. So very often number three would want to be sick because he wanted attention. I'm glad he's not a hypochondriac now because he used to want to be sick. He had asthma that was totally psychosomatic. 'Mommy, I have a temperature, I have a fever, I want to stay in bed.' Those were the symptoms. And number two would just go into himself, sit in his room and say that he didn't like or want to be with anybody, that being alone was his thing. So I guess those were the reactions.

"But, at the same time, I'm almost flabbergasted by the fact that the two of them, in spite of some jealousy, almost worship Dayem. You know how terrible he looked before his face operation. Yet, the other boys were not ashamed of him. On the contrary, they would follow him and do what he did. Maybe that's because they knew of the intense love that their mother has for him. If *he* can have the mother's love, then *we* will do the same thing to have the mother's love. But I don't want to go too deeply into psychology. The point is that Dayem has the complete love and trust of his brothers and that's a beautiful thing to watch that fills me with happiness.

"Now, because of all that he has learned about himself, Dayem is really not afraid of dying at all. He doesn't think he will, but if he does, he is certain that it will only be his body that dies. I've talked to him about this belief many times, and that's exactly where he is, and I am so happy for him because that's how I would want him to feel, how I would want myself to feel; but three or four years ago, it wasn't the case. He had a profound fear of death.

"I remember November 1983 so well. You had asked me to come to Children's to see Dayem and a psychologist. You had called me to tell me, 'It's better if you'd come because he's depressed.' So I came from wherever I was and stayed at the Children's Inn and was going to the hospital every day, and we were talking and talking about death and the body and the soul. He would say, 'I love life, I want to live.' And that was the most awful thing for me to hear, thinking that he was really at the end, and I didn't know by any means how to make him accept death. He didn't want to accept it. He refused it. But today he has made peace with it, which is absolutely marvelous—and it's particularly wonderful because he has accepted the idea, but no longer has the need. I've never seen him look so wonderful. Perhaps he will outlive all of us. And he will, in spirit if not in body."

W ORRY about your patient, my Brigham Hospital mentor, Dr. Samuel A. Levine, taught me. I do worry about Dayem, and I frequently find myself reflecting on his story. He is thirty-four now, and still actively pursuing his business deals, along with his brothers. His powerful bond with his mother continues as well, but he has had difficulty sustaining deep relationships with other women. He and the girlfriend of his thirtieth birthday remain friends, but they are no longer living together.

Dayem is always cheerful (at least to me) and his excellent heart function proves that he is taking his Desferal faithfully. He is at peace with his treatment, and I am no longer in a state of confrontation with him. But how long he will remain healthy, even with excellent compliance, I cannot know. I don't have enough experience with thalassemia patients over thirty to know what might befall him. It's likely, though, that I will celebrate the thirtieth anniversary of our first meeting. We are in the twenty-seventh year of our relationship now.

Will Dayem and my other patients with thalassemia go on to old age on their current regimen? I doubt it. There are too many risks involved with chronic red cell transfusion and intravenous catheters, and I have no idea about the toxicity of Desferal after multiple decades. So Dayem enjoys one year at a time. We try not to wring our hands about possible dangers. We know they are all around us, but he has decided to ignore them while I remain on watch. As a physician I must worry about threats to him that are within my power to deflect. As a patient, he must report unexpected events, but otherwise go on with his life.

When I crossed the bridge from the Brigham to the Children's nearly thirty years ago, Dr. Diamond told me that the greatest joy in pediatrics is to watch sick children shake off the fetters of chronic illness and become productive adults. He was, as usual, right on target. It is painful to see a chronically sick child. They are so helpless and innocent; they should be out playing with their friends instead of becoming battle-scarred veterans of medical technology. Hospitals, even fine ones like ours, are just not right for children. We do our best to offer them activities that may divert them, our superb nurses comfort them, and our wonderful housestaff of young interns and residents are desperate to cure them. But children should never see the inside of a hospital. We expect grandparents and even parents to get sick and require admission, but the times are out of joint whenever a child is encumbered by the trappings of a medical environment.

Therefore, whenever I confront a child with a chronic illness, I make a silent compact. I'm going to do everything I can to get that kid out of here and back to his or her family, and I'm not going to let the rules of biology stand in my way. If those rules won't let me succeed, I'll have to invent new ones; that's what clinical research is all about.

Is this just whistling in the dark to maintain my own morale? Is it merely the hubris of a competitive physician? Will I go too far in my zeal to breathe new life into a desperately ill child and thereby prolong pain and discomfort without realistic hope? I've seen all of these excesses in my day, but my job is to err on the side of over effort while, in each particular case, listening to the voices of those who say the child has suffered enough.

These very hard decisions about when to press on with technological interventions and when to acknowledge defeat are made particularly difficult today because of the speed with which advances are being made: we *can* win battles against biology in situations that would have been impossible only a few years ago. When Guido Fanconi advised Dayem's parents to avoid transfusion and let him go peacefully, he was right for that moment. But only a few years later, we learned how to administer Desferal, so that today, heart disease due to iron overload rarely occurs in patients who can comply with the treatment. Bone marrow transplantation was terribly dangerous when we began to develop our experience over twenty years ago, but now nearly 75 percent of patients with thalassemia who have compatible donors can be cured of their disease. If Dayem's heart fails again and cannot be corrected, we can even consider a heart transplant—a method of therapy that was certainly unavailable when Dr. Fanconi gave his advice.

I'm often asked whether it is right to go to the ends of the technological earth in an attempt to save or extend the life of one chronically ill child. The same health dollars, it is argued, could be spent on vaccinations that would prevent illness in thousands.

I find that a failed argument. As a physician, I am the advocate for my patient. If my patient wants to live and with his family is willing to enter the battle, it's my duty to take his hand and try to guide him through. My patients' hopes, and not the "sensible" use of the medical commons, have to be my fundamental goals. If my opinion runs counter to the views of advocates of cost control and resource utilization, I cannot help it. As long as I have a scientifically supportable reason to offer encouragement to a child, I must put that child's needs ahead of any broader consideration.

I am, in short, the servant of individual children. Only in such a role do I serve society as a whole. I have to admit, though, that I am grateful to be a pediatrician. It's much easier and more sensible to have such a view when children are patients. When we win back the life of a child, we gain decades of productive joy. Even if the cost is enormous, the gain is too great to measure. That is not true when patients are my age and older, and it is in the care of my age group that physicians find themselves caught in very serious ethical dilemmas.

Still, if physicians are mainly guided by the informed wishes of the patient and the practical application of technology, they are usually on firm ground. Theories of medical practice that focus on societal resources instead of the threat to an individual patient provide shaky underpinnings to medical care.

We have to remember, though, that technology itself is not the sole answer to serious illness. We physicians can't succeed unless our patients are full members of the health care team. For years I tried to persuade Dayem to take his Desferal regularly, and for years he evaded my every plea. I could do nothing for him until he made up his own mind to cooperate. By then it was almost too late. It is hard for a physician to admit that he or she is powerless. But we are, because we are only members of a care group, the central figure of which is the patient. The sense of omnipotence that many young physicians feel as they master abstract diseases disappears rapidly in the clinic and on the ward, as they gain experience with patients, each of whom is uniquely human.

Life in research is much harsher now than it was when I first moved to Children's Hospital, and the fabric of medicine is changing for the worse as profit motives make an unseemly entrance. Yet I cannot imagine a happier and more fulfilling profession. To this day, fascinating patients and their families inspire me to dream of far-off lands and challenge me to find answers where there were none. And some of the finest teachers, colleagues, and young investigators known to medical science have locked arms with me over the years in trying to meet those challenges. Yes, there are still huge inequities in health care delivery and gross inadequacies in modern medicine's ability to heal. But if I could turn back the clock and start again, I would walk through the same doors, and look down the same hallway, hoping to catch another glimpse of a boy called Immortal Sword.

Further Reading

Bothwell, T. H., J. T. Cook, and C. A. Finch. *Iron Metabolism in Man*. Oxford: Blackwell Scientific, 1979.

Bunn, H. F., and B. G. Forget. *Hemoglobin: Molecular, Genetic and Clinical Aspects*. Philadelphia: W. B. Saunders, 1986.

McDonagh, K. T., and A. W. Nienhuis. "The Thalassemias," in D. G. Nathan and F. A. Oski, eds., *Hematology of Infancy and Childhood*. 4th ed. Philadelphia: W. B. Saunders, 1993.

Modell, B., and V. Berdoukas. *The Clinical Approach to Thalassemia*. London: Grune and Stratton, 1984.

National Heart, Lung, and Blood Institute. *Cooley's Anemia: Progress in Biology and Medicine*. A review of the current status of activities in basic and clinical research in Cooley's anemia and recommendations for the future. Washington, D.C.: U.S. Department of Health and Human Services, 1987.

Orkin, S. H. "Diseases of Hemoglobin Synthesis: The Thalassemias," in G. Stamatoyannopoulos, A. Nienhuis, P. Leder, and P. Majerus, eds., *The Molecular Basis of Blood Diseases*. Philadelphia: W. B. Saunders, 1987.

Platt, O. S., and G. J. Dover. "Sickle Cell Disease," in D. G. Nathan and F. A. Oski, eds., *Hematology of Infancy and Childhood*. 4th ed. Philadelphia: W. B. Saunders, 1993.

Watson, J. D., and J. Tooze. *The DNA Story*. San Francisco: W. H. Freeman, 1981.

Weatherall, D. J. "The Thalassemias," in G. Stamatoyannopoulos, A. Nienhuis, P. Majerus, and H. Varmus, eds., *The Molecular Basis of Blood Diseases*. Philadelphia: W. B. Saunders, 1994.

Weatherall, D. J., and J. B. Clegg. *Thalassemia Syndromes*. 3rd ed. Oxford: Blackwell Scientific, 1981.

Glossary

5-aza-cytidine An anticancer drug once used in the treatment of acute myelogenous and lymphocytic leukemia.

A gamma globin gene *See* gamma globin genes.

adenine One of two purine bases that are essential components of DNA and RNA. The other is guanine.

adult hemoglobin (hemoglobin A) The form of hemoglobin normally constituting virtually all of the hemoglobin of adults. It is composed of two alpha and two beta globin chains ($\alpha_2\beta_2$).

alkaptonuria Excretion in the urine of homogentisic acid, which causes the urine to turn dark on standing. The condition is due to an inherited deficiency of an enzyme called homogentisic acid oxidase.

allele One of two or more alternative versions of a gene. On a given pair of chromosomes, corresponding sites (loci) may be occupied either by two identical alleles (in which case the individual is said to be homozygous) or by two different alleles (heterozygous). Thus, a beta thalassemia gene is an allele of the beta globin gene on chromosome 11.

alpha globin chains The products of the alpha globin genes. They combine with beta chains to form adult hemoglobin ($\alpha_2\beta_2$) or with gamma chains to form fetal hemoglobin ($\alpha_2\gamma_2$).

alpha globin gene The gene that regulates the synthesis of alpha globin chains. The two alpha genes (one on each chromosome 16) switch on in the first weeks of gestation.

amino acid Any of a class of nitrogenous organic compounds that are essential components of proteins.

amniocentesis A procedure in which a needle with a syringe attached is inserted through the abdomen and into the uterus of a pregnant woman, to obtain amniotic fluid, usually for genetic analysis.

anemia A reduction below normal in the oxygen-carrying capacity of the blood, which occurs when the equilibrium between blood loss (through bleeding or destruction) and blood production is disturbed.

Anopheles mosquito A genus of mosquitoes, many species of which are vectors of malaria.

anticoagulant An agent that prevents or delays the coagulation of blood.

aplastic anemia A group of anemias, often accompanied by low levels of certain leukocytes (white cells) and platelets, in which the bone marrow is usually hypocellular and fails to produce adequate numbers of blood cells.

autoimmune disease Any of a group of disorders that result when an individual produces antibodies against constituents of his own tissues. Autoimmune diseases may be systemic (as in systemic lupus erythematosus) or organ-specific (as in autoimmune thyroiditis).

autotransplant A graft of tissue derived from another site in or on the body of the organism receiving it. Also called an autograft.

balanced polymorphism A steady state in the proportions of a population that have varying alleles of a given gene. This state of balance comes about when a mutation such as thalassemia confers some advantages over "normal genes" (in the form of protection from malaria in heterozygous individuals) and some disadvantages (in the form of early death in homozygous individuals and a lowered reproduction rate in heterozygous individuals). *See* **mutation.**

Banti's syndrome Spleen enlargement once thought to be caused by alcoholism, now known to be caused by obstruction of the splenic vein. Also called congestive splenomegaly.

beta globin gene The gene that regulates the synthesis of beta globin chains. The two beta genes (one on each chromosome 11) are expressed at a low level after eight weeks' gestation, but just before birth they rapidly increase their output to replace gamma chain synthesis. This is called the fetal switch.

beta globin chains The products of the beta globin genes. They combine with alpha chains to form adult hemoglobin ($\alpha_2\beta_2$).

beta mRNA The initial product of the beta globin gene. It is exported to the cytoplasm where it is translated by the protein synthesis machinery into beta globin chains.

beta plus thalassemia A form of beta thalassemia in which a small amount of normal beta globin chain is produced. Beta plus thalassemia genes markedly reduce but do not entirely abolish beta globin chain production.

beta thalassemia A form of thalassemia characterized by diminished synthesis of beta globin chains of hemoglobin. In the homozygous form (Cooley's anemia; Mediterranean anemia; thalassemia major), adult hemoglobin is virtually absent or greatly diminished and the disease becomes evident in the first six months of life. It is usually a severe disease, marked by anemia, an enlarged spleen, skeletal deformation, and an enlarged heart. In the heterozygous form (thalassemia minor or thalassemia trait), although adult hemoglobin synthesis usually is reduced by one half, the individual is asymptomatic, but there is sometimes moderate anemia and minimal enlargement of the spleen.

beta zero thalassemia A form of beta thalassemia in which no beta globin chains are produced.

bile pigment Any one of the coloring substances of the bile, including bilirubin.

bilirubin A greenish yellow compound derived from hemoglobin during the normal and abnormal destruction of red cells.

blood The fluid that circulates through the heart, arteries, capillaries, and veins, carrying nutriment and oxygen to the body's cells. It consists of a pale yellow liquid, the plasma, containing the microscopically visible elements of the blood: the erythrocytes, or red blood cells; the leukocytes, or white blood cells; and the thrombocytes, or blood platelets.

blood count The number of red blood cells, white blood cells, or platelets in a measured volume of blood, usually a cubic millimeter.

bone marrow The soft tissue that fills the cavities of the bones. The marrow is filled with fat and supporting cells in which the cells that produce blood cells proliferate.

bone marrow transplant A procedure in which a large needle with syringe attached is inserted into the pelvic bone of an anesthetized donor and about a pint of marrow cells and blood cells are sucked out. The cells are then given by vein to a compatible recipient who is suitably prepared to receive them. If all goes well, the donor marrow cells home to the recipient's marrow, where they grow into blood cells. In most marrow transplants, the donor and recipient must be immunologically compatible.

butyric acid A rancid-smelling short-chain fatty acid found in butter, sweat, feces, urine, and blood.

carrier A person who has one normal and one defective version of a given gene. A carrier is minimally affected by the defective gene but can pass it along to offspring. If the offspring inherit one defective gene from each parent, they will usually show signs of disease.

centrifuge A machine with a compartment that spins around a central axis in order to separate materials of different density, such as red cells and plasma.

chelator A drug used to treat poisoning from metals such as lead or iron.

chemotherapy The treatment of disease by chemical agents such as antibiotics and anticancer drugs.

chromium A blue-whitish, brittle metal whose radioactive isotope binds to red cells and can be used as a tracer of their survival.

chromosome A structure in the nucleus of cells containing a linear thread of DNA. Genes are sequences of DNA that are contained within chromosomes. Normally present in the somatic cells of humans are 46 chromosomes, including two (either X and Y in males, or X and X in females) which determine the sex of the organism. In the reproductive cells there are 23 chromosomes—an X in ova, and either an X or a Y in sperm.

codon A series of three adjacent bases in a strand of DNA or RNA that codes for a specific amino acid. Also called a triplet. *See* **genetic code.**

cDNA Complementary DNA. When an RNA sequence is copied by reverse transcriptase, the product is complementary DNA.

Cooley's anemia *See* **beta thalassemia.**

cytoplasm The part of the cell outside the nucleus.

cytosine A pyrimidine base that is an essential component of both DNA and RNA. *See* **thymine; uracil.**

DNA The molecule that carries genetic information for all organisms except the RNA viruses. DNA (deoxyribonucleic acid) consists of adenine, guanine, cytosine, thymine, deoxyribose, and phosphate.

DNA base sequencing A chemical procedure by which the linear array of the stream of bases in DNA is determined.

deferoxamine A chelating agent which binds with iron to form a soluble complex. *See* **Desferal.**

delta-beta thalassemia Thalassemia caused by a deletion of the delta and beta genes in the beta cluster on chromosome 11. The gamma genes upstream of the deletion seem to function at a higher than normal rate, yielding fetal hemoglobin. In the homozygous state, there is moderate anemia with 100 percent fetal hemoglobin.

delta globin gene A functionally unimportant gene just upstream of the beta gene on chromosome 11. It has many features of a beta gene, but it has a different base sequence that causes it to function at a very low level. Delta globin chains combine with alpha globin chains to form adult hemoglobin A_2 ($\alpha_2\delta_2$).

deoxyribose One of a class of sugars that contain five carbon atoms and an aldehyde group instead of oxygen. Along with purine and pyrimidine bases and phosphate groups, deoxyribose is a major constituent of DNA (deoxyribonucleic acid).

Desferal Trademark for the water-soluble mesylate salt of deferoxamine, used as an iron chelator. *See* **iron chelation.**

dominant gene A version (allele) of a gene that is expressed and affects the characteristics of an organism, regardless of the state of the corresponding allele.

E. coli *Escherichia coli*, a bacterium normally found in the intestinal tract of humans. *E. coli* is pathogenic when it escapes from the gut and enters the urinary tract or the blood.

electrophoresis The movement of charged particles suspended in a liquid, a gel, or on paper under the influence of an applied electric field.

enhancer A sequence of DNA to which enhancer-binding proteins adhere, switching on the transcription of DNA to mRNA.

enzyme A protein capable of greatly accelerating the chemical reaction of a substance (the substrate) without being destroyed or altered. Enzymes are often specific to a given substrate.

epsilon globin gene A beta-like gene on chromosome 11 that is expressed only very early in embryonic development. It is then switched off and is followed both anatomically and functionally by the G gamma and A gamma genes which produce fetal hemoglobin.

erythrocyte A red blood cell.

exon The parts of a structural gene that code for the mRNA of enzymes and structural proteins. Exons are separated from one another by introns (noncoding sequences of DNA). The entire gene (including exons and introns) is first transcribed into immature mRNA, and then the introns are spliced out to form the mature mRNA that is translated into protein in the cytoplasm.

expression *See* gene expression.

falciparum malaria The most serious form of malaria. It is caused by a protozoan in the blood and is transmitted from person to person by the Anopheles mosquito. *See* **malaria.**

ferroxamine The red compound formed when iron is chelated by deferoxamine.

fetal hemoglobin The form of hemoglobin composed of two alpha and two gamma globin chains ($\alpha_2\gamma_2$). It makes up most of the hemoglobin in the fetus and is minimally present in adults. In aplastic anemia, leukemia, sickle cell anemia, and homozygous beta thalassemia fetal hemoglobin is variably elevated. Also called hemoglobin F.

fetal switch The process whereby the activity of the gamma gene is replaced by that of the beta gene when the fetus is nearly ready for birth. *See* **beta globin gene.**

fetoscope An endoscope for viewing the fetus in utero.

founder An individual in whom a mutation of a gene in sperm or egg cells arises spontaneously.

G6PD Glucose-6-phosphate dehydrogenase, an enzyme which protects red cells from oxidant damage. When G6PD is deficient, severe red cell damage may occur if certain drugs such as antimalarials are ingested.

G gamma gene *See* gamma globin genes.

gallstone A solid mass, usually made of cholesterol and more rarely of bilirubin, formed in the gallbladder or bile duct which may block the duct and can cause both jaundice and excruciating pain.

gamma-delta-beta thalassemia Thalassemia caused by deletion of the A and G gamma, the delta, and the beta globin genes on one copy of chromosome 11. Infants with this inherited defect are born with severe anemia because the gamma genes on the unaffected chromosome 11 are unable to keep up with hemoglobin demand during fetal life. After the fetal switch is completed (around six months of age), the anemia subsides.

gamma globin chains The products of the gamma globin genes. They combine with alpha chains to form fetal hemoglobin ($\alpha_2\gamma_2$).

gamma globin genes Two very similar but not identical genes on chromosome 11 (called A gamma and G gamma) which are active in fetal life, producing gamma globin chains. Gamma genes are switched off after birth, and their activity is replaced by the switching on of beta genes before birth.

gene The unit of heredity. It consists of a sequence of base pairs in the DNA molecule which controls the synthesis of one particular protein or RNA molecule. Each gene is located at a specific place on a specific chromosome.

gene expression The process by which genetic information is converted into mRNA molecules and then into proteins.

gene replacement therapy The insertion of a normal gene into tissue cells to replace a defective gene.

genetic code The 64 codons (nucleotide triplets) of messenger RNA and the 20 amino acids they specify. All but two of the amino acids can be specified by more than one codon, but each codon can specify only one amino acid. Three codons, called "stop" codons, do not specify any amino acid but rather terminate protein synthesis.

genetic engineering The manipulation of DNA in the laboratory to generate new combinations of genes or new DNA sequences. Often used synonymously with the term "recombinant DNA techniques."

genome The genetic material of an organism.

genotype An organism's genetic information. *See* **phenotype**.

gerocytes Old red cells in the circulation. Normal red cells live between 100 and 120 days.

globin The protein constituent of the hemoglobin molecule, which takes the form of four globin chains (two alpha and two beta chains in the adult).

globin synthesis rate The rate of production of globin chains. Usually assayed by measuring the incorporation of radioactive amino acid into globin chains.

glutamic acid An amino acid found in all in proteins. It is the number 6 amino acid in the beta chain of globin. In sickle hemoglobin, it is replaced by valine.

graft-versus-host disease A severe disease which results when a graft (such as a bone marrow graft) contains immune cells that attack the tissues of the recipient (host) because they are nonidentical to the graft cells. Clinical symptoms include skin rash, severe diarrhea, and liver dysfunction. The disease is often fatal but sometimes can be controlled with immunosuppressive drugs. Tissues capable of inducing graft-versus-host disease include the spleen, lymph nodes, thoracic duct lymph, the bone marrow, and blood.

granulocytes A class of leukocytes that ingests bacteria.

guanine One of two purine bases that are essential components of DNA and RNA. The other is adenine.

heme A nonprotein, insoluble iron compound found in hemoglobin, various other respiratory pigments, and many cells, both animal and vegetable. It is responsible for the characteristic coloring and oxygen-carrying properties of hemoglobin. There is one heme bound to each of the four globin chains of hemoglobin.

hemoglobin The oxygen-carrying protein in red cells. It contains four heme groups and four chains of globin which, together, can bind oxygen in the lungs and release it in the tissues. *See* **adult hemoglobin; fetal hemoglobin**.

hemoglobin A Adult hemoglobin.

hemoglobin F Fetal hemoglobin.

hemophilia A hereditary disease characterized by spontaneous or traumatic hemorrhage under the skin; from the mouth, gums, lips, tongue, and urinary tract; and into the joints and muscles. An X-linked recessive trait, it affects males, while females are carriers and only rarely affected.

hemorrhage The escape of blood from the vessels. Bleeding.

hepatitis Inflammation of the liver.

heterozygote An individual possessing two different versions (alleles) of a given gene. When a heterozygous person has one defective and one normal gene but is himself or herself minimally affected by the defective gene, that person is said to be a carrier. In thalassemia, the heterozygous person is said to have thalassemia trait.

homozygote An individual possessing two identical versions (alleles) of a given gene.

homozygous beta thalassemia *See* beta thalassemia.

hormone A chemical substance produced in the body by an organ or cells of an organ which has a specific regulatory effect on the activity of other organs. Examples are insulin and thyroid hormone.

hydroxyurea An agent used in the treatment of chronic myelocytic leukemia because it inhibits cell division.

immune *or* **immunity cells** Small lymphocytes called T or B lymphocytes. T cells undergo a maturation process in the thymus, which confers resistance to infectious diseases caused by certain bacteria, fungi, and viruses. They are also responsible for certain aspects of resistance to cancer, for delayed hypersensitivity reactions, for some autoimmune diseases, and for graft rejection, and they play a role in certain allergies. B cells produce antibodies under the control of T cells.

immunosuppressive drugs Drugs that suppress the action of T and B lymphocytes, antibody production, and sometimes the actions of scavenger cells such as macrophages.

intramuscular Within a muscle.

intrinsic factor A protein secreted in the stomach necessary for the absorption of vitamin B_{12}. Lack of intrinsic factor results in pernicious anemia.

intron Noncoding sequences of DNA within structural genes. Introns are transcribed into mRNA along with exons, but are spliced out prior to translation. *See* **exon.**

intron mutation One of six broad subtypes of mutation in the globin genes which can cause thalassemia. An intron mutation severely inhibits (but usually does not entirely abolish) the process whereby introns are spliced out of mRNA. Since some beta globin chains are usually produced, it is usually a beta plus mutation.

iron chelation The removal of iron from the body through the use of a drug that binds iron. The iron-containing compound is then excreted in the urine.

iron deficiency An inadequate level of iron in the body.

iron metabolism The absorption, utilization, and excretion of iron.

iron overload A condition in which the body contains excess iron. At high levels, the excess iron leads to oxidant damage throughout the body and can severely injure the heart, pancreas, liver, and other organs if it is not removed, usually through iron chelation.

irradiation Treatment which bombards target tissues with photons, electrons, neutrons, or other ionizing radiation in order to inhibit cell replication.

kidney Either of two organs in the lumbar region of the abdomen that filter the blood, excreting the end-products of body metabolism in the form of urine and regulating the concentrations of hydrogen, sodium, potassium, phosphate, and other ions in the extracellular fluid.

kilobase 1000 bases in DNA and RNA. The length of a gene is measured in kilobases.

leukemia A progressive, malignant disease of the marrow, spleen, and lymph nodes, characterized by uncontrolled proliferation of leukocytes (white blood cells) in the blood and bone marrow.

leukocyte A white blood cell.

liquid scintillation counter An instrument for indicating the emission of weakly ionizing particles, making possible the determination of the concentration of radioactive isotopes in the body or other substance. The radiation is absorbed by a phosphor crystal, which emits minute flashes of light that are detected and amplified by a photomultiplier tube.

lymphocyte A particular type of white blood cell (leukocyte) formed in the lymph nodes, spleen, tonsils, and thymus. These immunity cells make up approximately one quarter of all leukocytes in the blood of normal adults. *See* **immune cells.**

lysine An amino acid widely distributed in proteins.

malaria An infectious febrile disease caused by protozoa of the genus *Plasmodium*, which are parasitic in the red blood cells and are transmitted by the bites of infected mosquitoes of the genus *Anopheles*. The disease is characterized by attacks of chills, fever, and sweating occurring at intervals which depend on the time required for development of a new generation of parasites in the body. After recovery from the acute phase, the disease has a tendency to become chronic, with occasional relapses.

Mediterranean anemia Beta thalassemia.

mRNA Messenger RNA, a type of RNA which transmits information from DNA to the protein-forming system of the cell.

moiety Any equal part. A half. Also any part or portion.

molecular medicine Medical diagnosis and treatment using genetic techniques.

mutation A spontaneous or induced change in the DNA sequence of a gene in an individual organism. Mutations occur with high frequency, and are usually harmless. Others can lead to serious disease or disability. When a particular mutated gene provides the organism with an adaptive advantage, it will tend to be passed along to subsequent generations and to accumulate in the population. When a particular mutated gene is detrimental to the survival and reproduction of the organism in which it arises, it may lead to abortion or early death or to a lowered rate of reproduction. *See* **balanced polymorphism.**

myoglobin The oxygen-transporting pigment of muscle, composed of one globin chain and one heme group (containing one iron atom).

neocyte The newly formed and therefore the younger population of red cells. *See* **gerocyte.**

neocyte-gerocyte exchange The exchange of old red cells in a patient for young red cells from a donor through transfusion.

nonsense mutation A mutation which produces a nonsense codon (that is, a codon that does not encode any amino acid and which stops protein synthesis) in the place where a normal codon should have been.

nucleus The membrane-bound part of animal and plant cells which contains the chromosomes.

nucleated Having a nucleus or nuclei.

nucleated red cell A red cell with a nucleus.

nucleotide A compound composed of a base (purine or pyrimidine), a sugar (ribose or deoxyribose), and a phosphate group. DNA and RNA are made up of nucleotides.

organelle A membrane-bound organized living particle present in practically all eukaryotic cells. Types of organelles include mitochondria, Golgi complexes, endoplasmic reticula, lysosomes, and ribosomes.

ossicle A small bone, especially one of the three bones of the inner ear.

outbreeding Mating between unrelated individuals.

pernicious anemia An anemia occurring in children but more commonly in later life, characterized by malabsorption of vitamin B_{12} due to a failure of the gastric mucosa to produce intrinsic factor.

phagocyte Any cell that ingests microorganisms or other cells and foreign particles. In many cases the ingested material is digested within the phagocyte.

phenotype An organism's observable characteristics. *See* **genotype**.

pigment gallstone A gallstone made of bilirubin.

plasma The pale yellow fluid portion of the blood in which the particulate components are suspended.

plasmid Any extrachromosomal self-replicating element of a cell. In bacteria, plasmids are circular DNA molecules that reproduce themselves and are thus conserved, apart from the chromosome, through successive cell divisions. Plasmids may also become integrated into the bacterial chromosome and are sometimes called episomes. Plasmids frequently confer resistance to antibiotics.

platelet A disk-shaped structure found in the blood of all mammals which plays a major role in blood coagulation. Platelets are formed in the marrow, lack a nucleus and DNA, but contain active enzymes.

pneumococcal pneumonia An acute febrile disease produced by the streptococcus pneumoniae and marked by inflammation of one or more lobes of the lung, together with consolidation.

pneumococcus An individual organism of the species *Diplococcus pneumoniae*.

point mutation A mutation resulting from a change in a single base pair in one gene in the DNA molecule.

polymer Any compound of high molecular weight consisting of up to millions of repeated, linked units.

polymerase Any enzyme that catalyzes the process by which simpler molecules are combined to form a larger molecule (called a polymer).

polymerase chain reaction (PCR) A method by which individual genes or stretches of DNA can be numerically amplified.

polymorphism The state of being in several different forms. *See* **balanced polymorphism**.

porphyria Any of a group of disturbances of porphyrin metabolism, characterized by marked increase in formation and excretion of porphyrins or their precursors. Heme is a porphyrin.

prenatal diagnosis Diagnosis of a condition in the fetus.

prognostic groups Groups of patients with a certain disease who have different estimated survival times based on findings at the time of diagnosis.

promoter The region of DNA just "upstream" of a gene to which certain proteins, called transcription factors, bind and which position other proteins, called polymerases, to initiate transcription of the gene.

prostaglandins Chemically related long-chain fatty acids that stimulate uterine contraction and lower blood pressure. They have several other important functions as well.

protein synthesis In organisms other than viruses, the complex process whereby genetic information contained in the DNA is first transcribed into mRNA inside the cell nucleus and then translated into an amino acid chain on the ribosomes in the cytoplasm.

purine An organic base. Adenine and guanine are purine constituents of DNA and RNA.

pyridones A class of compounds that chelate iron.

pyrimidine An organic base. Thymine and cytosine are pyrimidine constituents of DNA. Thymine and uracil are pyrimidine constituents of RNA.

recessive gene A gene that produces an effect in an organism only when an identical allele of the gene is inherited from both parents, that is, only when the individual is homozygous for that gene.

recombinant DNA DNA that has been constructed in the laboratory using various genetic engineering techniques.

recombinant DNA techniques *See* genetic engineering.

recombination The process by which one or more nucleic acid molecules are rearranged to generate new sequences of DNA.

Recombinant DNA Advisory Committee (RAC) A standing committee of the National Institutes of Health with oversight responsibilities for the use of recombinant DNA in laboratories and in clinical applications.

red cell One of the elements of the blood, an erythrocyte. Normally, in humans, the mature form is a nonnucleated, biconcave disk, adapted, by virtue of its configuration and its hemoglobin content, to transport oxygen.

red cell transfusion Administration to a patient of red cells obtained from a donor.

regulator gene A gene whose product is a protein that regulates the transcription of one or more structural genes.

repressor A transcription factor that binds to a particular domain of DNA and reduces or halts the transcription of a gene.

incorrect →

restriction The process of splitting DNA into fragments through the use of restriction enzymes. Restriction occurs naturally among bacteria, and is used by scientists in the laboratory to chop up DNA into analyzable pieces.

Failure of viruses to "reproduce" in certain bacterial strains, Due to Restriction

restriction enzyme Any of the natural and synthetic enzymes that *enzymes.* catalyze the splitting of DNA into fragments.

restriction fragments DNA that has been chopped into pieces smaller than the DNA molecule, with the use of restriction enzymes.

reticulocyte A young red blood cell which still contains RNA that forms threads in the cell with certain stains.

retrovirus A large group of RNA viruses that invade animal cells and are responsible for a wide range of animal diseases, including anemia, malignant tumors, and leukemia. In humans, retroviruses cause AIDS and certain rare leukemias.

reverse transcriptase An enzyme of retroviruses that catalyzes the transcription of the viral RNA to DNA, which is then incorporated into the genome of the host cell.

Rh disease An anemia that begins in fetal life when antibodies generated by the mother cross the placenta to enter the fetal circulation and destroy fetal red cells. Also known as erythroblastosis fetalis.

ribosome The RNA-containing particle (organelle) in the cytoplasm active in the synthesis of protein.

RNA A nucleic acid found in all living cells. In its various forms, RNA (ribonucleic acid) is involved in all stages of protein synthesis, as well as in many regulatory and catalytic roles. In certain viruses, RNA constitutes the viral genome. It consists of adenine, guanine, cytosine, uracil, ribose, and phosphoric acid.

SCID *See* severe combined immune deficiency.

severe combined immune deficiency An inherited disorder of the immune system characterized by loss of cellular immunity and antibody production. Also known as SCID.

shunt In the context of thalassemia, a surgically created union of two blood vessels.

sickle cell anemia A hereditary, genetically determined anemia caused by a single mutation in the beta globin gene. In the United States it is observed almost exclusively in blacks and, in homozygous individuals, is characterized by bone pain, acute abdominal pain, ulcerations of the lower extremities, anemia, and sickle-shaped red blood cells. Also known as sickle cell disease.

sickle cell trait Heterozygous sickle cell anemia, usually asymptomatic.

sickle hemoglobin (hemoglobin S) An abnormal hemoglobin in which there is a substitution for the amino acid glutamic acid in the number 6 position of the beta chain by valine. Hemoglobin S changes its shape to an elongated or sickle form when oxygen is withdrawn.

Southern blot A method, named after its inventor Edward Southern, by which DNA restriction enzyme fragments, one or more of which may contain a specific gene, are separated from one another in a semi-solid matrix such as a gel through which an electric current is passed and subsequently overlaid with a probe of radioactive cDNA that is "complementary" to the specific gene and binds to it. This identifies that the gene is present in the DNA fragment mixture and measures the size of the DNA restriction fragments in which the gene resides.

spleen A large organ about the size of a flattened orange situated in the upper left part of the abdominal cavity. It produces lymphocytes and cleans the blood of aged or deformed blood cells. It also clears the blood of particles such as bacteria.

splenectomy Surgical removal of the spleen.

splenomegaly Enlargement of the spleen.

stem cell A rare cell in the bone marrow whose descendents multiply and specialize into all the mature cells found in the blood, including red cells, white cells, platelets, and lymphocytes.

streptococcal sepsis Blood stream invasion by streptococci. Usually a very serious disease.

subcutaneous Beneath the skin.

structural gene A gene whose product is a structural protein. *See* Regulator gene.

synthesis The combining of separate elements to form a whole.

thalassemia A heterogeneous group of hereditary anemias which have in common a decreased rate of synthesis of one or more hemoglobin polypeptide chains and are classified according to the chain involved (α, β, γ, δ). The two major categories are alpha thalassemia and beta thalassemia. It is manifested in homozygotes by profound anemia or death in utero, and in heterozygotes by relatively mild red cell anomalies. *See* **thalassemia intermedia**.

thalassemia intermedia Thalassemia which clinically appears to be intermediate between homozygous and heterozygous beta thalassemia.

thalassemia major Homozygous beta thalassemia. *See* **beta thalassemia**.

thalassemia minor Beta thalassemia trait.

thalassemia trait Heterozygous thalassemia, manifested by relatively mild red cell anomalies.

thrombocyte A blood platelet.

thymine One of two pyrimidine bases that are essential components of DNA. The other is cytosine. *See* **uracil**.

titrate To adjust a substance to a precise level.

transcription The process whereby the sequence of bases in DNA is encoded into a strand of mRNA. Transcription is the first step in protein synthesis.

transcription factors Proteins in the nucleus that act as enhancers, repressors, or promoters.

transferrin Serum protein that binds and transports iron.

transfusion The introduction of whole blood or blood components directly into the blood stream.

translation The process whereby information encoded in a strand of mRNA is used to produce a protein. Translation occurs on the ribosomes in the cytoplasm.

transplant To transfer tissue from one part to another. An organ or tissue taken from the body for grafting or infusion into another area of the same body or into another individual.

tRNA Transfer RNA, a type of RNA which, during protein synthesis, matches amino acids to their codons on mRNA.

urea A small molecule produced in the liver that is the chief waste product of body nitrogen and is excreted in the urine.

uracil One of the two pyrimidine bases of RNA. The other is cytosine. *See* **thymine**.

white cell A leukocyte. A cell in the blood which ingests particles or performs immune functions such as cellular immunity, antibody formation.

Wiskott-Aldrich syndrome An immunodeficiency syndrome caused by the inherited deficiency of a specific protein. The disease is transmitted as an X-linked recessive trait. The condition is characterized by chronic eczema, chronic infections, bleeding, and anemia.

zeta gene A primitive hemoglobin gene expressed very early in embryonic life. It is analogous to the alpha gene.

Index

Abortion, 10, 140, 141, 181; selective, 140, 146, 152, 153, 189, 192; public opposition to, 142–143; by women with thalassemia trait, 144, 146, 147, 149; caused by prenatal diagnosis, 148, 153–154; fetal research and, 150–151

Adult hemoglobin. *See* Hemoglobin A

AIDS, 16, 45, 161, 162, 190

Alkaptonuria, 25, 26

Alpha globin gene(s): chains, 29, 30, 32, 33–34, 69, 70, 71, 72, 93, 135, 175, 189, 194; chromosome location, 31, 70; mutations, 33, 70; unmatched, unpaired, 69, 70, 71, 72, 194–195; precipitates, 71, 93; production of (synthesis), 135, 189; fetal hemoglobin produced by, 137; radioactive, 145, 162; presence, absence of, in thalassemia, 164–165; mapping, 176, 177; base sequences, 177

Alpha thalassemia, 70–72, 137, 189; gene character, presence, absence in, 164, 165, 178–179

Altay, Cigdem, 179, 180

Alter, Blanche, 148, 152, 153, 179

Amine groups, 99

Amino acid, 25, 26, 28, 156–158; in protein, 14, 27, 165; substitution, 27–29, 30, 33–34, 159; sequence, 29, 30, 33, 155, 159, 165; in hemoglobin chains, 33; radioactive, 60–62, 63, 140, 181; chains, 158; encoding, 158

Amniocentesis, 154, 188

Anemia, 5, 59; accompanying thalassemia, 6, 7, 8, 13, 14, 29, 56, 60, 66, 70, 137, 195; heart failure accompanying, 7, 11, 13; severe, 13, 14, 187; red cell production and appearance, 14, 48, 67, 68; mild, 16, 179; pernicious, 42, 43; congenital, 53; splenectomy for, 60. *See also* Sickle cell disease

Animals used in research and experimentation, 79, 110, 111–112, 116, 117, 199

Anopheles mosquito, 18, 19, 201

Antibiotics, 42, 79, 95, 214, 224; broad spectrum, 91, 92, 95; effect on pregnancies, 143; resistance to, 166, 167, 168

Antibodies, 90, 92

Anticancer drugs, 197–198, 199, 209

Antileukemia drugs, 198, 199, 208

Ascorbic acid (vitamin C), 101, 102, 104

Avery, Oswald, 24, 165–166

Bach, Fritz, 82

Bacteria, 90, 91–92, 95, 119, 165, 172; enzymes in, 47, 188; iron required by, 98–99; protein in, 163; resistant, 166–167; used in gene cloning, 167–169

Bacteriophages/phages, 163

Baltimore, David, 160–161, 162, 163, 169

Bank, Arthur, 182

Banti, Guido, 54–55

Banti's syndrome, 54, 55

Bauer, Walter, 53

Beadle, George, 26, 29, 158
Beardsley, Peter, 199
Beecher, Henry, 64
Benz, Edward, 160, 162, 197
Berg, Paul, 167
Berlin, Nathaniel, 46–47
Beta globin gene(s), 7–8, 210;
    production of hemoglobin by, 12,
    34, 50, 52, 69; chains, 28, 29, 30, 32,
    33–34, 51, 56, 58, 69, 70–71, 72,
    135, 136, 138, 140, 144, 159, 160,
    175, 178, 186, 194, 195;
    chromosome location, 31, 137, 138,
    175, 196; mutations, 33, 152, 153,
    159, 165; in thalassemia, 34, 35, 55,
    66, 137, 139, 152, 195; precipitates,
    71; unmatched, unpaired, 70–71,
    72; injection into bone marrow,
    119–120; production of (synthesis),
    135, 136, 138, 140, 144, 163,
    173–175, 181, 186, 195; /gamma
    chain ratio, 140, 141; radioactive,
    140–141, 144, 145, 161, 162;
    presence, absence in DNA, 164, 177,
    180, 181, 182; cloning, 168, 185;
    composition (coding blocks),
    173–175; mapping, 176–177, 178;
    base sequences, 177, 185; failure to
    switch on at birth, 195
Beta thalassemia, 20–22, 58, 69, 71,
    73, 152, 160, 185; severe, 51–52,
    60, 70, 145; genetic/genes, 55–56,
    57, 164; fetal hemoglobin
    production in, 56, 62, 182; beta
    plus type, 59, 136, 178, 179, 185,
    186, 187; beta zero type, 59, 136,
    177, 178, 182, 183, 184, 185, 186,
    187; fetal, 137; trait, 139, 145,
    152, 179; homozygous, 152; cause
    of, 163, 182–183, 186, 187;
    molecular basis of, 178, 182;
    nondeletional, 183
Biology, molecular, 114, 139, 154,
    158, 160, 179, 197, 210
Blackfan, Kenneth, 74
Blood: genetic diseases, 59, 73, 160,
    173; infections, 91–92, 95; banks,
    153. *See also* Fetus/fetal: blood
    samples; Red blood cells;
    Transfusion
Bone fractures, 10, 14, 16, 50. *See
    also* Saif, Dayem: bone fractures,
    and risk of
Bone marrow, 12, 82, 85–86, 207; red
    cell production in, 5, 6–7, 9, 12, 13,
    14, 43, 46, 60–61, 77, 78, 119, 139,
    195–196, 197, 198, 199, 202, 208;
    rubbish-eating cells in, 14, 69–70,
    135–136; iron in, 35; volume,
    expansion, 49–50, 96; injection of
    beta globin genes into, 119–120;
    insertion of retroviruses into, 192;
    stem cells, 195–196
Bone marrow transplantation, 78, 80,
    81; for leukemia, 33, 133, 208–209;
    for thalassemia and other blood
    diseases, 77–78, 79, 80, 82, 84–85,
    86–87, 194, 208–209, 210; graft
    failure, rejection of transplanted
    cells, 77, 78, 79, 80, 85, 208, 210;
    compatible donors for, 78, 80, 82,
    83, 85, 87, 132, 194, 208, 248; risks
    and fatality rates, 78, 80–81, 82,
    83–87, 132–133, 134, 248;
    autotransplants, 208–209. *See also*
    Graft-versus-host disease
Brenner, Sydney, 156
Butyric acid, 200, 206–207

Cancer, 45, 46, 48–49, 50, 104, 198,
    209. *See also* Chemotherapy
Cao, Antonio, 152, 153
Castle, William B., 26–27, 43, 73, 74
Cell(s), 18, 90, 209; immune system,
    43, 82, 208; stem, 82, 195–196,
    209, 210; walls, membrane, 99,
    194; rubbish-collecting, 105;
    cytoplasm, 156, 157, 158;
    decoding by, 162; protein
    production in, 175–176; division,
    199. *See also* Platelets; Red blood
    cells; White blood cells
Centrifuge process, 5, 49, 214
Chang, Henry, 151
Chargraff, Erwin, 24
Chelators/chelation, 99, 102, 110,
    118, 129, 136, 210; iron overload
    and, 100–101, 106, 108, 109, 116;
    oral iron, 108–109, 116, 120, 121,
    194, 207, 226; adverse effects of,
    117, 120; toxicity of, 120, 121
Chemotherapy, 46, 208, 209
Chromosomes, 161, 166, 171;
    location of genes on, 23–24, 29,
    30, 31, 32, 166, 176
Ciba-Geigy Pharmaceutical
    Company, 99, 108–109, 110, 116,
    117
Cividalli, Gabriel, 144
Clegg, John, 53, 72, 135

Clinical trials/investigations. *See* Research: clinical
Codons, 157, 158, 159, 175, 184, 185, 186
Complementary DNA (cDNA), 167, 168, 175, 184, 188; radioactive, 162–163, 164, 178, 180, 183; beta, 183
Conflict of interest issues, 63–64. *See also* Ethics, medical
Cooley, Thomas B., 6, 53, 189
Cooley's anemia. *See* Beta thalassemia
Cooley's Anemia Foundation, 194
Corner, George W., 53–54
Crick, Francis, 24, 155
Cytidine, 197–198, 199
Cytoplasm, 156, 157, 158

Dacie, John, 204
Darwin, Charles, 20
Deferroxamine. *See* Desferal
Delta-beta thalassemia trait, 179, 182
Delta globin gene(s), 31, 137, 138, 180, 181, 182
Desferal, 99, 107–108, 117, 119, 153; intramuscular injections, 100, 101, 102, 116, 130, 233; oral, 100, 108–110, 116; intravenous drip, 102–103, 213, 214, 222, 247; subcutaneous pump delivery, 103–106, 107–108, 120, 121, 122–123, 128, 129, 130, 132–133, 144, 193, 212–213, 218, 219, 221, 222, 233–234; adverse effects of, 104, 106–107, 109; age of patient and, 106–107, 120–121; cost of, 108–109, 193; shunt delivery, 213, 214, 215, 217, 218, 219, 221–222, 234, 242. *See also* Saif, Dayem: Desferal treatment; noncompliance
Diabetes, 42, 101, 102, 103, 104; children of mothers with, 200, 203, 206
Diamond, Louis K., 50–51, 52, 55, 57, 59, 67, 73, 74, 76, 204, 247
DNA, 34, 47, 164; double helix shape, 24, 25, 155, 157, 164; nucleotide bases, 24, 25, 155, 156, 157, 158, 186; fetal, 154, 180–181; research, 156, 163, 169–172, 173; TAG in, 158; viruses, 161, 163; base sequencing, 163–164, 165, 175, 176, 184, 188; substitution,

165, 184–185; chromosome locations, 166; enhancer domains, 176, 196, 203; prenatal diagnosis by, 177; loading, 180; drug therapy and, 197, 198–199. *See also* Complementary DNA; Recombinant DNA
Drug(s): antimalarial, 67; immunosuppressive, 78, 80; therapeutic, 80, 114–115, 136, 195; companies, 108, 109, 110–111, 114; research, 110–111, 119; clinical trials, 118–119, 121; dumping, 119–120; corticosteroid-like, 126; illegal, 131; resistance, 167; for fetal hemoglobin production, 195, 203; anticancer, 197–198, 199, 209; antileukemia, 198, 199, 208; to manipulate fetal switch, 200; cost of, 207; cardiac, 214, 223, 226. *See also* Antibiotics

Edelin, Kenneth, 140, 142, 153
Ehrlich, Paul, 79
Enders, John, 75
Enhancers, 176, 196, 203
Enzymes, 25–26, 156, 160, 161, 167, 188; production of (synthesis), 26, 166, 176; in bacteria, 47, 188; restriction, 47, 163–165, 167, 178, 185; transcription by, 156, 157
Epsilon globin genes, 31, 32, 176, 196
Escherichia coli, 92, 166
Ethics, medical, 249; issues in research and experimentation, 64, 115–116, 118–119, 184; peer review system, 120; influence on technology, 146; standards, 146–147. *See also* Abortion; Research: fetal, ethical issues and debates
Exons, 175, 196

Falciparum malaria, 19, 20, 21. *See also* Malaria
Faller, Douglas, 200, 206, 207
Fanconi, Guido, 8–9, 10, 12, 13, 97, 187, 248
Ferrebee, Joseph, 79, 80
Ferroxamine, 99, 100
Fessas, Phaedon, 71, 72, 152
Fetal Research Law, 149–150
Fetoscope, 148, 151, 152, 153, 179, 180–181

Fetus/fetal: blood samples, 148–149, 151, 154, 179, 180–181, 189; switch (fetal to adult hemoglobin production), 177, 192, 195–196, 199, 200, 202, 206–207. *See also* Abortion; Hemoglobin F (fetal hemoglobin); Research: fetal, ethical issues and debates; Thalassemia: fetal; prenatal diagnosis of
Finch, Clement, 78, 80
5-aza-cytidine, 197–198, 199
Fogerty, John, 41, 42
Forget, Bernard, 75, 136–137, 138, 154, 160, 162, 164, 182, 183, 184
Frei, Emil, 46
Freireich, Emil, 46
Frigoletto, Frederic, 148–149

Gabuzda, Tom, 60, 61, 62, 63
Gallbladder, 49, 53
Gamma-delta-beta thalassemia, 139, 182
Gamma globin gene(s), 52, 177; fetal hemoglobin production in, 12, 196, 198; chains, 32, 34, 56, 66, 70, 72, 135, 136, 138, 139, 140, 144, 182, 195, 196, 197, 199, 203; in thalassemia, 35, 56, 59, 66, 137; production of (synthesis), 135, 136, 137, 138, 140, 182, 195, 197, 199, 203, 206; chromosome location, 138; radioactive, 145; A gamma, 176, 181; G gamma, 176; base sequences, 177; on and off switching, 198; expression, 207
Gamma thalassemia, 137
Gardner, Frank, 59
Garrod, Archibald, 25, 29
Gene(s): hemoglobin, 7, 19, 52, 134, 173; thalassemia, 18–19, 20, 26, 55–56, 173; pools, 19, 33; chromosome locations, 23–24, 29, 30, 31, 32, 166; dominant, 23; recessive, 23; coding, coding blocks, 24–25, 158, 175; absent, deleted, 26, 164–165, 178–179, 180, 185, 189; enzyme production in, 26; regulation, 34, 176; function, 38; transfer/replacement therapy, 46, 87, 136, 165–166, 177, 194, 195, 208, 210; cloning/replication, 165, 166, 167–169, 172, 185, 186, 187, 188, 192, 210; resistance, 167, 168;

base sequencing, 173, 175, 176, 177, 185, 186; structure, 173, 196; stability, 175; expression, 176, 207; splicing, 186, 187. *See also* Globin gene(s); Mutation(s)
Genetic(s), 8, 23–24, 38, 152–153, 170–171; medical, 26, 141; hemoglobin, 29–30; immunologic compatibility in transplantation, 79, 80; molecular, 136, 192, 204; outbreeding, 152
Gerald, Park, 59, 60, 71, 171
Gerocytes, 214, 219, 225. *See also* Transfusion
Gilbert, Walter, 165
Globin gene(s), 33, 176; chains, 135, 136, 138, 140, 149, 151, 177, 195; chromosome location, 138, 139; deletion, 139; mRNA production in, 160, 162; on and off switching, 196. *See also* Alpha globin gene(s); Beta globin gene(s); Epsilon globin gene(s); Gamma globin gene(s); Zeta globin genes
Glutamic acid, 28, 33, 34, 159
Graft-versus-host disease, 78, 82, 86, 134, 208; symptoms, 81, 133; autotransplantation and, 209
Granulocytes, 121
Griffey, Susan, 179, 180, 181
Gunn, Robert, 71, 72

Health care system, 44–45, 113, 114, 190, 193, 249
Heart: disease, 7, 11, 13, 15, 16, 36, 37, 83, 89, 90, 98, 125, 193; iron overload and, 15, 16, 101, 102, 104, 105–107, 108, 214, 248; enlargement of, 50; muscle damage, 221; transplantation, 248
Hematology, 8, 78, 120; experimental, 46, 139, 197; pediatric, 73, 74; research, 135, 141
Heme, 23, 28, 29, 30, 175
Hemoglobin: as oxygen carrier, 5, 6, 14–15, 30, 70, 159; deficiency, 5, 12, 13, 16, 48; genes, 7, 9, 19, 23–24, 27, 29, 31, 32–34, 52, 134, 173; iron and, 14–15, 23; mutations/abnormalities, 26, 27, 29, 33, 34, 38, 48, 67–68, 159, 201, 203; sickle cell, 27, 29, 33, 34; composition of, 29, 70; production of (synthesis), 29, 51; evolution, 30–31, 32;

Hemoglobin *(continued)*
   clinically silent, 33; research, 50,
   134; levels in red blood cells,
   55–56, 57, 89, 137; precipitates,
   68, 69, 70, 71; solubility of, 68;
   unbalanced synthesis of, 71, 72,
   194
Hemoglobin A (adult hemoglobin),
   5, 55; presence, absence in
   thalassemia, 12, 34, 52, 56, 58, 60,
   187; production of (synthesis), 12,
   32, 34, 50, 52, 69, 175, 194;
   absence of, in sickle cell disease,
   27, 29; chemical composition, 29,
   30, 32; survival rate, 61, 62, 66. *See
   also* Fetus/fetal: switch
Hemoglobin F (fetal hemoglobin), 5,
   31, 32, 55, 138–139; presence in
   thalassemia, 12, 34, 50–52, 56, 57,
   58, 60, 67, 136, 179, 207;
   production of (synthesis), 12, 34,
   50–51, 56, 62, 70, 72, 135–136,
   137, 144, 176, 182, 194, 195, 197,
   198, 199, 206–207; in red blood
   cells, 13, 60, 61, 69, 197, 206–207;
   percentage of total hemoglobin,
   52, 196–197; survival rate, 61, 62,
   66; hereditary persistence of
   (HPFH), 182; sickle cell disease
   and, 199–200, 202–203; ethnic
   demographics, 201–203. *See also*
   Fetus/fetal: switch
Hemoglobin H, 71
Hemophilia, 22–23
Hepatitis, 15–16, 35
Herrera, Miguel, 36, 77, 83, 89, 90,
   95, 96
Herrick, James, 6
Heterozygotes, 178, 180, 188. *See
   also* Thalassemia: trait
Hill, Lister, 41, 42
Hitzig, Walter, 8
Hobbins, John, 180–181
Holley, Robert W., 158
Homozygotes, 178, 179, 180, 181
Hormones, 13–14, 16, 42, 220, 236,
   237
Housman, David, 160, 164, 183, 184
Huehns, Ernest, 144
Hydroxyurea, 198–199, 200, 203, 207

Identical twins, immunologic
   compatibility of, 78, 80, 82
Immune system, 20, 35, 83, 161;
   cells, 43, 82, 208; immunologic

compatibility and, 78, 80, 82;
   bone marrow transplants and,
   80–81, 84, 86; inherited diseases
   of, 81–82, 83. *See also* AIDS
Immunosuppressive drugs, 78, 80
Inducers, 175
Informed consent, 63, 64, 88, 112
Ingram, Vernon, 29, 33, 34
Inherited disease(s), 9; research, 22,
   23, 45–46; treatment, 22, 23, 210;
   of the blood, 59, 73, 160, 173; of
   the immune system, 81–82, 83; of
   bone marrow, 85. *See also*
   Thalassemia; Sickle cell disease
Inhibitors, 175
Intrinsic factor, 43, 73
Introns, 175, 186, 187, 196
Iron, 5, 15, 48; in transfused red blood
   cells, 8, 126, 214; hemoglobin and,
   14–15, 23; in globin chains, 29; in
   bone marrow, 35; levels in red
   blood cells, 48, 49, 67, 100; bacteria
   required by, 98–99; -binding plasma
   protein, 98; toxicity, 98, 133;
   deficiency, 99, 100; salts, 99–100;
   balance, 100, 103, 116, 126;
   excreted in urine, 100, 102–103,
   104, 105, 106, 116–117, 125–126,
   133; absorbed by intestine, 104;
   storage pools, 105, 106, 107, 126,
   133
Iron overload, 215; as result of
   transfusion, 8, 14, 15, 35, 83, 95,
   98, 103, 126, 214; risk of death
   from, 8, 16, 35, 98, 125; adverse
   effects of, 15, 101, 102, 103, 106,
   108; heart disease resulting from,
   15, 16, 101, 102, 104, 105–107,
   108, 214, 248; as result of bone
   marrow transplantation, 84;
   chelation treatment for, 100–101,
   106, 108, 109, 116. *See also* Desferal
Irradiation. *See* Radiation
Isotopes, 60–62, 63
Itano, Harvey, 27–29

Jacob, François, 156, 175–176
Janeway, Charles A., 73, 74
Jaundice, 48, 49, 53, 90, 133
Jefferson, Mildred, 142
Jones, Chester, 48, 52, 54, 55

Kan, Alvera (nee Limauro), 75, 138,
   141
Kan, Debbie, 138, 139

Kan, Yuet Wai, 73, 75, 137, 138, 140, 141, 152, 164, 182–183, 184–185
Kazazian, Haig, 185–186, 187
Keberle, Heinrich, 99, 100–101, 109, 110
Khorana, H. Gobind, 158
Kidneys, 13–14, 78–79, 117, 132

Lantigua, Cathryn, 229
Lasker, Mary, 41, 42
Leder, Philip, 173
Lee, Pearl, 53
Letvin, Norman, 199
Leukemia, 46, 80, 81, 82, 84, 86; bone marrow transplantation for, 33, 133, 208–209; drugs to prevent, 198, 199, 208
Levine, Samuel A., 69, 88–89, 246
Limauro, Alvera (married name Kan), 75, 138, 141
Linch, David, 199
Liquid scintillation radioactivity counter, 61–62, 161
Liver, 6, 39, 47, 54–55; enlargement of, in thalassemia, 6, 7, 12, 90, 98; rubbish-eating cells in, 14, 70, 136; iron overload and, 15, 101, 102, 106
Lodish, Harvey, 160
Loukopoulos, Dimitris, 152, 153
Lymphocytes, 208

Mahoney, John, 151
Malaria, 19, 20, 21, 22, 33, 51, 67; gene mutations as protection from, 18, 19, 20, 201, 203
Malpractice suits, 88
Maniatis, Tom, 177–178
Mathé, George, 77
Maxam, Allan, 165
McCaffrey, Ron, 162
McClintock, Barbara, 175, 176
Means, James Howard, 53
Medical schools and teaching hospitals, 39, 40, 42, 43, 44–45, 190, 205
Mediterranean anemia. *See* Thalassemia
Mendel, Gregor, 23, 26
Meningitis, 92, 129, 235
Messenger RNA (mRNA), 156–158, 160, 161, 162, 166, 173, 175; alpha, 164; beta, 164, 165, 183, 184, 186; production of (synthesis), 176, 183, 186; failure to function, 183, 184, 185
Miller, Barbara, 202–203, 206, 207
Modell, Bernadette, 144
Monod, Jacque, 175–176
Mullis, Kary, 188
Murray, Joseph, 125, 126–127, 128, 130
Mutation(s), 19, 27, 28, 34; of thalassemia gene, 20, 22, 182, 183, 185–186, 189, 201, 209; of hemoglobin gene, 26, 27, 29, 33, 34, 38, 48, 67–68, 159, 201, 203; point, 28, 159, 165, 182, 185, 186–187, 189; of alpha and beta chain genes, 33, 186, 187; nonsense, 184–185, 186; beta zero, 186

Nathan, Jean, 228, 230
Nathans, Daniel, 47, 163, 167
National Institutes of Health (NIH): research funding and facilities, 39, 42–44, 45, 65, 66, 75, 112, 154; rules and review boards, 64–65, 119; Recombinant DNA Advisory Committee (RAC), 169, 171
Neel, James, 26, 27, 29
Neocytes, 214, 219, 225. *See also* Transfusion
Neveska, Josephine, 51, 67–68, 69
Nielands, John, 98–99
Nienhuis, Arthur, 197
Nirenberg, Marshall, 158

Olivieri, Nancy, 120–121, 207
Operators, 176
Organ transplantation, 78–79, 80
Orkin, Stuart, 139, 180, 181, 182, 185–186, 187
Ottolenghi, Sergio, 182
Oxygen: in hemoglobin, 5, 6, 14–15, 30, 70, 159; in lungs and tissues, 29, 32, 38; in muscles, 31; /carbon dioxide exchange, 33

Pancreas, 15, 101, 106
Parasite, malaria, 18, 19, 20
Patton, Dorothy, 229
Pauling, Linus, 26–29
Penicillin, 42, 64, 91–92, 95
Perrine, Richard, 201–202
Perrine, Susan, 200–201, 203, 204, 206, 207
Peter, Heinrich, 109–110, 116, 117
Phages, 163

Phagocytes, 90
Physician: /patient relationship, 65–66, 115, 130, 215–216, 241; salaries, 65, 66, 205; role in treatment decisions, 87–88; secondary (financial) gain from treatments, 115–116; specialists, 190
Plasma, 5–6, 49, 98, 207, 242
Plasmid, 166–167, 168
Platelets, 82, 208, 219, 242
Platt, Orah, 200
Pneumococci pneumonia, 42, 92, 165–166
Polio, 75, 149
Polymerase chain reaction (PCR), 187–189
Polymerases, 24
Polymorphisms, 20, 33
Porphyria, 23
Promoters, 176, 186, 196, 203
Propper, Richard, 102, 103
Protein, 12, 155–156, 161; amino acids in, 14, 27, 165; production of (synthesis), 24, 38, 70, 155, 156–157, 160, 166, 173, 175; chains, 29; intrinsic factor, 43, 73; composition of, 156–158, 159; in bacteria, 163; nuclear, 195–196; enhancer-binding, 196. *See also* Enzymes; Red blood cells

Radiation, 77, 78, 79, 80, 208. *See also* Alpha globin gene(s); radioactive; Amino acid: radioactive; Beta globin gene(s): radioactive; Complementary DNA: radioactive; Gamma globin gene(s): radioactive; Liquid scintillation radioactivity counter
Recombinant DNA, 119, 165, 167, 169; gene cloning, 24–25, 156, 162, 166–167, 188; for thalassemia, 136, 139; research, 169–172, 173
Recombinant DNA Advisory Committee (RAC), 169, 171
Red blood cells, 7, 43, 48; defective, misshapen, 5, 6, 12–13, 14, 66–67, 68, 90, 93; deficient hemoglobin levels in, 5, 12, 13, 16, 48; destruction of, 5–6, 7, 12, 71, 91; nuclei/nucleated, 5, 6–7, 13, 48, 60, 137, 139; production (synthesis) and development of, in bone

marrow, 5, 6–7, 9, 12, 13, 14, 43, 46, 60–61, 77, 78, 119, 139, 195–196, 197, 198, 199, 202, 208; iron levels in transfused blood, 8, 126, 214; fetal hemoglobin levels in, 13, 60, 61, 69, 197, 206–207; thalassemia trait, 20, 207; debris, rubbish in, 48, 66, 67, 68; iron levels in, 48, 49, 67, 100; G6PD enzyme in, 67, 68; staining of, 67–68, 69; hemoglobin precipitates in, 68, 69, 70, 71; membrane, 69, 71; globin chain production in, 135, 136, 137, 138, 140, 149, 151, 177, 195; fetal, 145, 181, 206; mRNA molecules in, 160. *See also* Hemoglobin; Transfusion
Repressors, 176, 196
Research, 45, 47–48, 83, 113–116, 120, 149, 154, 190–191, 204; clinical, 39–40, 41–42, 44, 45–46, 63–64, 86–87, 104, 118–119, 145, 247; funding, 39, 41, 43–44, 45, 59, 64, 72, 110–111, 112–113, 114, 172, 184, 205; biomedical, 41, 66; competition, 45–46, 117–118, 184, 205–206; hematology/hemoglobin, 50, 134, 135, 141; thalassemia, 53, 54, 60, 63–64, 172, 176–187, 190, 194; drug, 110–111, 116–117, 119–120; indirect costs of, 111–113, 114; gene, 119, 155, 169–170, 204; fetal, 140, 143, 149, 150–151, 153–154; fetal, ethical issues and debates, 141–143, 147, 148–151, 152–153, 154; DNA, 156, 163, 169–172, 173
Retroviruses, 161–162, 192, 210
Reverse transcriptase, 161, 162, 184
Ribosomes, 157, 158, 160, 184–185, 186
RNA, 161–162, 166. *See also* Messenger RNA; Transfer RNA
Roe v. Wade, 141–142
Rosen, Fred, 81

Saif, Dayem: enters treatment, 1–2, 11, 35; physical appearance, 1–2, 3, 5, 93–94, 97, 98, 122, 123, 212, 214–215, 217, 220, 230, 232; symptoms and diagnosis, 5–6, 8, 12, 13, 90, 136; bone fractures, and risk of, 10, 36, 93, 95, 96–97, 131, 231; heart condition, 11, 13, 36, 89, 90, 98, 132, 213, 214–215, 217, 220, 221–223, 224, 226, 246, 248; personality, 11–12, 18, 89, 127–128,

211, 219–220; blood transfusion therapy, 13, 16, 18, 35, 36, 37, 83, 84, 89–90, 93, 95, 96, 126–127, 129, 132, 136, 212, 213–214, 217, 225; removal of spleen, 13, 90–91, 92–93, 95, 124, 136, 219; life and treatment in Mexico, 35–36, 77, 89–90, 95–96, 232; risks of treatment, 37, 83, 92–93, 95; as candidate for bone marrow transplantation, 83, 84, 132–133; annual reevaluations in Boston, 96, 105, 122–123, 129, 223, 225; deafness, 96, 97; iron accumulation, 97, 98, 101; Desferal treatment, 101–102, 105, 122–125, 128–134, 136, 155, 211–214, 217–224, 226–227, 233–234, 242, 246, 249; lifestyle and personal relations, 123, 124, 125, 128, 129–131, 213, 218, 219, 220, 226, 227, 235, 236–237, 246; plastic surgery, 123–124, 125, 126–128, 130; noncompliance, 215, 218, 221, 226, 245, 249; mental health, 215–216, 217, 234, 242; hormone replacement therapy, 220, 236, 237; thirtieth birthday, 227, 228–230; philosophy of life, 237, 238–240, 242

Saif, Mr. (father), 3, 9, 18, 37, 128, 225, 235, 239

Saif, Mrs. (mother), 221–222, 230, 231, 239; appearance, personality, ethics, 2–3, 94–95, 146, 147, 243, 244; guilt about Dayem, 9, 18, 37; children born after Dayem, 10, 245; dedication to Dayem, 37, 222, 243, 244–245; risks of Dayem's treatment and, 37, 91, 92–93, 124; reports on Dayem from Mexico, 77, 89–90, 96; participation in treatment program, 95, 101–102, 130, 233

Saif, Mssrs. (brothers), 10, 225, 230, 245, 246

Salaries, medical, 40, 44, 59, 65, 66

Salvarsan ("606"), 79

Sanger, Fred, 165

Schwartz, Eli, 75

Severe combined immune deficiency (SCID), 81

Shannon, James, 41–42, 43–44, 47

Sharp, Philip, 173

Shurin, Susan, 102

Sickle cell disease, 6, 27–29, 33, 34, 141, 159, 176, 185; bone marrow transplantation for, 85, 209; trait, 141, 201, 202, 203; genetic coding for, 159, 185; fetal and adult hemoglobin production and, 199–200, 202–203; environmental conditions and, 201–202, 203; drug therapy for, 203, 207

Smith, Hamilton, 163, 167

Sociobiology (Wilson), 170

Southern, Edward/Southern blot method of analysis, 164, 165, 178, 179, 180, 181, 182, 189

Spleen: enlarged, in thalassemia, 5, 6, 7, 12, 54–55, 60, 67, 90; red blood cells and, 6, 68–69; removal of (splenectomy), 13, 55, 60, 67, 68–69, 71, 90, 91, 92, 136; rubbish-eating cells in, 14, 68, 69–70, 90, 91, 135–136

Stem cells, 82, 195–196, 209, 210

Tatum, Edward, 26, 29

Temin, Howard, 160–162, 163

Testosterone, 220, 236, 237

Thalassemia, 14, 33, 53–54, 183; Mediterranean origin of, 2, 6, 8, 19, 34, 53, 54, 140, 152, 153, 185–186, 187, 189; hemoglobin levels in, 7, 49, 60, 71, 82, 144, 162; physical deformities caused by, 7, 106; life expectancy and, 8, 19–20, 22, 51–52, 84, 87, 125, 153; severe, 8, 19, 26, 29, 34, 51, 55, 57, 135, 141, 143, 149; evolution of, 18–22, 28, 29, 34, 35, 51, 54, 55, 57, 58, 71, 159, 160, 163, 173, 176, 177, 178, 185; trait, 19, 20, 22, 27, 29, 33, 51, 54, 57, 143, 144, 148, 178, 181; gene mutation, 20, 22, 182, 183, 185–186, 189, 201, 209; mild, 26, 51, 55, 70, 72, 135; treatment (general discussion), 29, 36–37, 62, 155, 190, 194, 203, 207; symptoms and diagnosis, 34, 48–49, 51, 139–140; cure, anticipated, 35, 82, 172, 209–210, 248; molecular basis of, 47, 102, 135, 173, 178, 187, 189; in adults, 49, 52; intermedia, 50, 51, 52, 58, 60, 72, 207; imbalance concept in, 71, 72–73; globin chain production in, 135; fetal, 137–138, 139–140, 141, 143, 144–145;

Thalassemia *(continued)*
  prenatal diagnosis of, 139–140,
  141, 143, 144, 145–146, 147, 148,
  151, 152–153, 154, 172, 177, 179,
  180–181, 185, 188–189, 192;
  prevention, 147, 207. *See also*
  Bone marrow transplantation;
  Research; Transfusion
Thomas, E. Donnall, 77, 78, 80, 81,
  84, 125
Toxic poisoning, 98, 99, 120, 121, 133
Transcriptase, reverse, 161, 162, 184
Transcription, 156, 157, 186, 196,
  203
Transfer RNA (tRNA), 157, 158, 160
Transfusion, 70, 91, 93, 137, 153,
  214; iron overload caused by, 8,
  14, 15, 35, 83, 95, 98, 103, 126,
  214; as treatment for thalassemia,
  8, 9, 13, 14, 49, 51–52, 87, 97, 98,
  106, 136, 144, 190, 210, 220; risks
  of, 13, 15–16, 35, 83, 84, 247;
  bone marrow transplantation and,
  84; donors, 214; neocyte-gerocyte
  exchange, 214, 219, 225
Transplantation, organ, 78–79, 80.
  See also Bone marrow
  transplantation
Tuan, Dorothy, 182
Tumors, 161–162, 209

University hospitals and research
  facilities, 110–111, 113, 114,
  115–116

Urine, 25, 26, 49, 90, 100, 198; red
  (iron excretion), 100, 102–103,
  104, 105, 106, 116–117, 125–126,
  133

Vaccines, 75, 92, 149, 248
Valentine, William, 26
Verma, Inder, 162
Viral infections, 91–92, 149
Virology, 149, 161, 162, 169
Virus(es): polio, 160; AIDS/HIV, 161,
  162; DNA, 161, 163, 166, 173;
  RNA, 161. *See also*
  Bacteriophages/phages
Vitamin(s), 5, 42; B_{12}, 42, 43, 73; C,
  101, 102, 104

Waldmann, Thomas, 47
Walzer, Stanley, 171
Watson, James, 24, 155
Weatherall, David, 53, 54, 72, 135,
  182, 198, 202
Weissman, Sherman, 47, 178,
  182
Whipple, George, 53–54
White, Paul Dudley, 53
White blood cells, 82, 119, 208
Wilson, Edward O., 170–171
Wintrobe, Maxwell, 26
Wiskott-Aldrich syndrome (WAS),
  81–82, 84

Zeta globin genes, 31, 32
Zubrod, Gordon, 40–41, 46